Karl-Heinz Rauscher

# Energy Medicine
## Healing Voices Rainbow

**Shamanic Healing & Symptom Constellations**

BoD - Books on Demand
Norderstedt

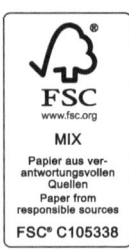

Bibliographic information of the German National Library:
The German National Library lists this publication in the German National Bibliography; detailed bibliographic data can be found on the Internet at http://dnb.dnb.de.

© 2024 Dr Karl-Heinz Rauscher
www.dr-rauscher.de
Translation of the German original, ISBN: 978-3-7578-2981-0
The work, including all its parts, is
protected by copyright law. Any use not authorised by the author is prohibited. This also applies to distribution by radio, television, photomechanical reproduction, sound storage media of any kind, the reprinting of extracts as well as the
storage and processing in electronic systems.
Translation into English: Andrew Swift
Proofreading: Margaret Swift
Portrait photo: Melanie Jeanne Ann Wagner
Cover and typesetting: Karl-Heinz Rauscher
Cover image: "human-meditate-mind": Benjavisa Ruangvaree
with licence from Shutterstock.com ID: 1886209099

Publisher: BoD · Books on Demand GmbH,
In de Tarpen 42, 22848 Norderstedt
Printed by: Libri Plureos GmbH, Friedensallee 273, 22763 Hamburg

ISBN: 978-3-7597-8450-6

For all

# Table of contents

# Foreword

Energy is the magic word. Everything in our living world is energy. Life itself is energy. We as human beings are filled with energy; our bodies are created and maintained by energetic processes.

An understanding of this basic reality is still alien to modern Western medicine, the reason being the historical intellectual fixation on visible and measurable matter, a fixation that came about as a reaction to the authoritarian interpretation of the world by religions.

The separation of matter and spirit by the philosophers of the Enlightenment overcame the dominance of religion in popular thinking and established modern science, which limits its perception of nature to the five senses. As a result, scientists of that era considered only matter which could be recognised through pure observation as worthy of investigation. The spirit, and thus all invisible, non-measurable energetic processes, were tainted by association with religion. The rationally minded wished (and still wish) to avoid falling into the clutches of religions whose leaders believed themselves entitled to dictate to scientists what is allowed and what is not. The taboo on the scientific investigation of spiritual and energetic processes is a direct consequence of the collective trauma stemming from the witch hunts and burnings which went on over centuries and ensnared anyone, male or female, who thought differently. It is a millionfold trauma that persists to this day, is firmly embedded in our society and leads to a heightened level of fear in the collective unconscious. Behind the rejection of spiritual-energetic healing powers by many scientists lies the unconscious fear of being ridiculed, banished from civil society and ultimately put to death. Because these processes take place within the collective subconscious mind, people are unaware of them. The rejection of energetic healing is an automatic response, a collective reflex that bypasses the mind. Reflex responses can, however, only be justified in situations of immediate danger. Later, when the danger has passed, and especially when the time comes to analyse the natural world scientifically, with dispassionate intellect, such automatic responses have no place. Because at this point, they rob us of our reason.

The continued existence of this reflex indicates that the danger is not yet emotionally over, that many people living today are still collectively so traumatised in their deepest souls by the millionfold slaughter in the Middle Ages that they cannot see reality and the forces at work in it. We suffer from a collective, post-traumatic psychosyndrome in which unconscious fear leads to the suppression of common sense and, as a result, to total ignorance of natural, energetic phenomena. The result is a distorted view of nature. A fundamental barrier has thus been set up in the scientific world, which prevents the observable from being investigated.

In rejecting all spiritual, energetic processes in the human body and soul, conservative scientists make a twofold mistake. On the one hand, they reject spiritual connections so as not to expose themselves to religious authoritarianism and, unconsciously, to deadly persecution. On the other hand, they adopt the same automatic condemnation of all spiritual healing from the monotheistic religions which demonised such spiritual healing powers as manifestations of the indigenous nature-based religions that were to be eradicated and whose healer practitioners were to be burned at the stake, drowned or simply hanged from the nearest tree.

In this way, the entire Western scientific world has adopted the very belief system that it actually wanted to move away from and into which it is determined not to fall back under any circumstances, come hell or high water. Because it is a completely unfounded belief that energetic-spiritual forces do not exist or, if they do exist, that they only cause evil and harm people.

As long as matter had not yet been researched to the last detail and its exploration continued to produce new, valuable findings, even without the assumption of a spiritual background, this was not so bad. However, since matter has now largely revealed its secrets and even DNA, our genetic code, has been deciphered to the last building block, research into life's mysteries is no longer making any real progress. We are going round in circles.

Since we were presented with the indisputable findings of quantum physics, which prove that matter breaks down into something that has never been associated with matter, namely energy and connection – all of this under the gaze of physicists – it should be clear to everyone that, in order to better understand life, we need to expand our framework of understanding. The invisible world of energy and the relationships between the energetic units now comes into consideration. For this to happen, Western science would have to abandon once and for all the belief that the invisible does not exist and is therefore not worth investigating. It is a belief that is nothing more than a religious dogma which should no longer have any place in scientific thinking.

If only a third of the world's research funds – many billions – were invested in clarifying the energetic background to the phenomenon of life, we would soon have proof of what the doctors and healers of this world who work with healing energies have known for a long time based on their own experience:

Matter is generated by energy and sustained in its existence by energy. Energy permeates the entire universe and connects all its parts into a functioning whole. There are energetic structures that can not only maintain order in the universe and all its parts, including the human body and the human psyche, but also restore it in the event of disruption. In addition to the energetic forces that maintain life in its healthy functions, there are however also energetic interference fields that lead to illness and pain. Most interesting for medicine is the fact that healing energies also exist. Similar to the earth's magnetic field, they are present everywhere, are totally geared towards recovery and have the power to heal physical illnesses and also mental disorders, or at least to make a significant contribution to healing.

This book is intended to open the eyes of my medical colleagues, of the scientific community and of all people who are interested in the background of life to the highly interesting world of energy which forms the basis of life, which permeates all of us completely and to which we owe our existence. But the most positive aspect is that these energy worlds contain forces that are able to heal us on all levels.

This book is my legacy as a doctor to the world.

# Introduction

Exploration of the invisible is the great adventure of the future. It is an adventure, because we do not know what lies ahead of us. The new and unknown is inconceivable within the old thought patterns, cannot be grasped with the familiar linguistic terms and cannot be measured with the instruments we have had at our disposal up to now. It transcends our horizons. Just as, in the Middle Ages, the realisation that the earth is round literally lay 'beyond the horizon', and we first had to venture to the edges of the then known world in order to prove a truth already recognised in theory, so today we too must venture to the edges of our imagination and sail beyond until new land appears and makes a new kind of understanding possible. This will give us insights into the truths of living nature that are still hidden today.

We know from history that it is not easy for people to abandon the fixed framework of thought to which they have adhered throughout life, only to realise that the world as they conceived it up to now does not exist, indeed has never existed.

But the spirit of enquiry, which is an important characteristic of our species, has always led us beyond the current horizon. So come with me on a journey to new horizons, beyond which we will discover together how the astonishing phenomena of energy medicine can be explained and what new picture of existence emerges from them.

Albert Einstein, one of the most intelligent thinkers of the modern era, was inspired by the view beyond this very horizon to write the following words:

"Everything is energy and that's all there is to it. Match the frequency of the reality you want, and you cannot help but get that reality. It can be no other way. This is not philosophy. This is physics."

Einstein's realisation that everything is energy confirmed the idea I already had as a medical student that there is a deeper reason, a deeper cause behind the body – namely matter – and that doctors can only understand the illnesses of their patients when they recognise the energy structure that underpins and conditions this body and therefore also its illnesses.

The great inertia of old thought patterns is reflected in the fact that hardly anything has changed in medical research to this day – even post-Einstein and in the face of the quantum physical evidence for his findings. Medical researchers still cling to the traditional, material view of the human body and refuse to take the experiences of shamanic healers and energy medicine practitioners of modern times seriously, failing to recognise them as perceptible, natural phenomena. However, such recognition is precisely the prerequisite for utilising the enormous potential of this planet's creative spirit of research and the enormous financial resources that flow into medical research worldwide for research into energetic phenomena of the body and soul.

As a specialist in internal medicine, a family constellator and now also a shamanic healer, I have experienced countless examples which today make it certain to me that energetic processes are not only the cause of physical and mental illnesses, but that they also play a leading role in the healing of those illnesses.

These experiences have brought me to the realisation that true healing is not possible without the contribution of the energy worlds that surround us and in which we live. Energy medicine understands the energetic connections, researches them more closely and incorporates them into the treatment of patients. It has the potential to revolutionise the future of medicine. Shamans throughout all eras and on all continents use energetic healing methods. In addition, more and more doctors and healers around the world are discovering energy medicine. A wide variety of methods are being used.

In this book, I look forward to introducing you to two new and extremely effective methods of energy medicine: Symptom Constellations and the shamanic healing method known as 'Healing Voices'. The deeper backgrounds that emerge not only open up new healing possibilities, but also shed new light on the innermost core of the phenomenon of life.

Writing this book is an adventure for me, because I expect that I myself will come to new realisations and surprising insights during the writing process. I invite you to accompany me on the intellectual journey of this adventure.

## Chapter 1: The basics of energy medicine

"We are slowed down sound and light waves, a walking bundle of frequencies tuned into the cosmos. We are souls dressed up in sacred biochemical garments and our bodies are the instruments through which our souls play their music."
Albert Einstein

I owe my knowledge of energy medicine to my many years of experience with system constellations and the shamanic healing method known as 'Healing Voices'.

In order to understand the amazing healing power of energy medicine, I had to shake off the old thought patterns of the scientific world of our time and take a completely new mental path. In English, we speak of 'thinking out of the box' or, as Jens Corssen, a specialist in mental self-management, puts it, jumping out of the 'neuronal cot' and leaving the habitual thinking pathways of our brain behind to plunge into the daunting jungle of an unknown world.

I would like to describe the world that was revealed to me then right here at the beginning of this book, because it allows us to better understand and comprehend the healing phenomena of energy medicine.

### Energy worlds

We humans live within different energy worlds and energy levels that not only surround us, but also permeate every cell of our body and every layer of our aura. These energy worlds, which are organised in levels, in different qualities and frequencies, influence each other. They form an interconnected system, comparable to the earth's atmosphere, in which a change in one zone can soon lead to a change in the status quo of another, distant zone.

We are part of a larger context, a unity that can only be explained if we always keep the whole in mind. If, as is customary in Western science, we break the whole down into its individual parts and examine them under the microscope without making the connection to the whole, we miss the essential. As researchers, we are faced with a dilemma. Because the analytical mind can only understand by compartmentalising. In order to really grasp the whole, we would have to leave intellectual understanding behind and focus on a different kind of cognitive ability, namely the intuitive ability to perceive our entire being, including the body, soul and spirit. We would have to put out invisible antennae, not think but feel, be intuitively receptive, open ourselves to an insight derived from the big picture instead of seeking the solution by means of compartmentalisation.

Exploring the component parts makes perfect sense as long as we keep an eye on the whole and see and interpret the phenomena that we discover at the level of the smallest parts in the light of the whole. These two approaches will then complement each other; they belong together. However, we have to contend with the paradox that each part appears to be separate from other parts. This is the only reason why we are able perceive it as an independent part. But at the same time, the part is also the whole and, at this level, inseparably one with everything else. Both interpretations are true at the same time. It seems impossible to reconcile these two perspectives. But if we take the bold step to superimpose these two realities, like two slides showing the same object from different angles, then we see a completely different dimension. Our intuitive perception supports us in this endeavour.

In this book I want to take that bold step and look at the different levels of the energy worlds that surround us separately from each other, without losing sight of the whole. I hope that the insights arising from the intuitive perception of the holistic connections will thereby be rendered accessible to the analytical mind. In this way, the insights of energy medicine can enrich science and open up a new level of scientific research.

**Let's keep this always in mind:** The various energy qualities that surround us are closely interwoven. They form an all-connecting unity.

On this basis, I will now take a closer look with you at the various energetic qualities and show you how and where the greater whole affects the individual parts, including us humans.

First and foremost in this list are the generating energies that are able to create matter and do so continuously. Even if it is not clear at the moment why we need to know more about this if we want to understand the healing effects of energy medicine, we will encounter the generating principle again and again in this book on the way to a deeper understanding.

### Energies that generate

### The visible world of matter is generated by energy

What causes matter to exist is an old question. People throughout the ages have tried to find an answer to this question. We obviously find it difficult to live in a world that we cannot explain. The inexplicable frightens us. What we don't understand is threatening, simply because it might pose a threat. In the same way that an animal entering our cave in the dark is threatening as long as we don't know which animal it is. It could be a sabre-toothed tiger or just a sheep. We need to know so that we can protect the clan and the children from potential danger. So we thrust the torch of our knowledge into the darkness. Ah, just a sheep. All clear! Everyone can go back to sleep.

With regard to the forces that are behind matter and generate it, the luminosity of the torch of knowledge has not yet been sufficient to see what is really there. But we need to know. We need an answer. So people have always invented stories that gave the force behind matter a shape and a face. The creation myths were born. They gave our ancestors a sense of security.

We are unable to perceive the reality behind matter with our five senses, but we dearly wish to distinguish something on the white screen of the inexplicable. We have therefore simply inserted a film of the known, visible and tangible world into our projector and shown the images on the screen. This is why the creation myths of all eras are teeming with animals, snakes, birds, rams and bulls, or why a fatherly or motherly face appears to us from the screen of the unknown. Now, all we need to do is believe the stories we tell ourselves and we can feel safe in an uncertain world. Over time, we forget that we are – figuratively – sitting in a cinema and looking at an illusory world. Even after thousands of years, we still tell our children and grandchildren the same naïve stories so that they too can feel safe in an uncertain world.

These creation stories have nothing to do with reality. Even today, despite all scientific knowledge, we have to admit that we basically know nothing about the generative principle behind matter.

Modern science, which has developed precise measuring instruments to investigate matter, has on principle steered clear of the question surrounding the generation of matter and has been content to leave the subject to religious leaders because it did not want to deal with religious content. Science only asks "What is matter?" and not "Who or what created matter?".

But the question "What is matter?" was answered by quantum physics research decades ago. The answer is so astonishing and so 'out of the box' that the consequences have not yet been drawn in large parts of the scientific world, including medical research. The eminent physicist Prof Hans Peter Dürr, who was Director of the

Max Planck Institute for Physics and Astrophysics in Munich for many years, put it like this:

"Primarily (behind matter) there is only connection, the combining force that has no material basis. We could even call it 'spirit'."

When we look into matter using quantum physics methods and break it down to the last detail, it disintegrates before our eyes into an energetic force that creates connections or is itself a connection. Dürr explains it as follow: "There is only a structure of relationships, constant change, vitality."

The force or energy that creates this structure of relationships and thus matter is still unclear today. At this point, let us speak of the 'generating energies'. If the word 'energy' is already too specific, we can also speak of a 'generative principle'.

In order to understand and apply the effects of energy medicine, it is not important that we do not know more about the generating energies at the moment. What is important is that, at the base of all matter and therefore also of the human body, there are energetic, non-material connections that are in a constant state of change. This is the solid ground on which the proven and indisputable findings of quantum physics have placed us.

### Matter is a structure of energetic relationships that is in constant flux

Now that matter has been generated and we know that it is a constantly changing structure of relationships that connects us to the greater whole, we can turn our attention to the forces and energies that can affect and influence this structure of relationships that we perceive as 'matter'. This is exactly what we want to achieve in medicine – more specifically in energy medicine – to influence matter, for example to make a cancerous tumour disappear, to reduce an inflammation or to restore a damaged organ.

On the basis of what Dürr and other leading scientists have revealed, let us now abandon the conventional image of matter and realise that, even when we talk about people and their illnesses, we are always talking about energetic relationships. This makes it easier to understand what is really going on in the human body and psyche. Let us start from the whole picture, a context that works everywhere. Looking at the greater whole tells us (and this is logical at this level):

**If one part is sick, the whole is sick.**
**When one part becomes healthy, the whole becomes healthy.**

But before we go into detail here, let us familiarise ourselves with the other basic energy qualities to gain a better understanding. Let's take a look at a subarea first.

### Energies that sustain

Matter is sustained by the sheer existence of the energy that generates connection. The existence of matter is therefore linked to the existence of the connecting energy, to the simultaneous presence of energy and connection.

Thinking in the old scientific way means that we look at the parts in isolation from the whole and act as if it were possible for the part to be separate from the whole. This might lead us to believe that, once generated, the energy within the matter is sufficient to sustain it and that no further connection to the generating energy would be necessary. But that would be a mistake. For the connection is the second essential component of matter alongside the energy. Most important here is the connection of the part to the whole. It must not be neglected simply because it exists. This is why the idea that the part is separate from the whole is untenable. We would have a false picture of reality in front of us, an illusion.

The part is connected to the whole and therefore cannot exist without the whole, or more precisely, cannot sustain itself without the whole. It is therefore closer to the truth to imagine that the generating energy, which acts on the greater whole, sends energy impulses a million times a second (or infinitely many times a second) into the part of matter we are looking at in order to ensure the presence of the whole there. These continuous energy impulses sustain the matter. In this case, the generating energy also becomes a sustaining energy. Matter is regenerated every millionth of a second and thus preserved in its existence.

The urge of the analytical mind to differentiate between generating and sustaining clearly diminishes at this point. Looking at the whole, it is logical to say:

**For matter to persist, energy and connection are necessary at the same time.**

If we consider the greater whole (i.e. think holistically, think in a new scientific way), then whenever we look at matter, we are looking at energy which generates connection whilst at the same time also being this connection. When we look at our body, which consists of matter, we are looking at an entity that is connection and energy in all its parts and at the same time is generated and sustained anew every millionth of a second by this very energy, by these very connections. These energies connect us to the greater whole as well as to all its parts. We are deeply connected to nature, plants and animals and also to all mankind. This includes the people of earlier times, our ancestors, on whose existence our existence is based. Without the connections to our ancestors, we would not even exist. The timeless connections to the whole and its parts are the basis of our existence and therefore also the existence of our body.

**The body is energetically connected to the ancestors.**
**The energy of our ancestors is at work in our body.**

At this point it is clear that matter and therefore also diseased body cells can be influenced and also healed by changing the energy and the energetic connections. Influencing the energy quality and the quality of the connections tackles the root of the current problem and is a primary and therefore very effective healing method that permeates even the smallest cell structures.

**Energy medicine heals through intervention at the level**
**of energy and connections (relationships).**

Energy therefore generates and sustains matter with its connective quality. Even if it doesn't make sense from a holistic point of view (i.e. from a revised scientific point of view) to consider the connecting quality of energy in isolation from its other qualities, we still have to do so in order to take account of the old scientific way of thinking that we have all been so used to and that serves minds which can only understand through compartmentalisation. I don't know how long we will keep this up, but let's just continue to assume at this point that valuable insights can be gained by looking at what is separate because, after all, that is the assumption of all Western science. Of course, we will later integrate the insights gained in this way into the overall picture in order to gain a better understanding of reality. In this way, the holistic and the compartmental view might complement each other.

So let's take a closer look at the effects of the connecting energy.

### Energies that connect

The existence of connecting energies is shown by the fact that parts of nature regularly connect. There are examples of the effect of connecting energies on all levels:

29

## On a physical and material level

- A stone that falls to the ground

  It is connected to the earth by gravity, the nature of which is not yet understood.
  Of course, there must have been a separating energy beforehand, e.g. a person who picked up the stone and then dropped it. But we will come to the separating energies later, ... aha, so they are already at work here, the separating energies, because that which comes later is separated from the here and now. But only apparently, because from a holistic perspective, time also constitutes a unity. But, as I said, more on that later. However, we can already say that this separation is being cancelled out again with the help of the connecting energy of our consciousness. Consciousness? We will also come to that later.

- Two hydrogen atoms fuse in the sun to form a helium molecule

  The connecting forces here are heat and pressure. Again, we know that the driving energy behind them is gravity. The fact that gravity is not yet understood in its essence could indicate that there is another quality of energy behind gravity that has not yet been scientifically analysed. This could be the actual connecting energy.

- Air molecules (gases) mix in the earth's atmosphere and establish the closest possible and most varied contact with each other

  At this level, the connecting energies are the sun's heat and the earth's rotation. Temperature differences cause the air to circulate giving rise to winds and storms.

- The connection between oxygen and the body that comes about through the breathing process

  The connecting energy is a physiological necessity that triggers the breathing reflex. We breathe to avoid dying. The respiratory reflex is elementary for self-preservation. It connects us with air molecules and thus with the entire atmosphere of our planet. When breathing ceases, death occurs after a few minutes.

- Raindrops fall to earth and flow into the sea

  The water molecules of the fresh water mix with the water molecules of the sea and, in this way, create as close and free a connection as possible.
  Once again, gravity is the connecting energy. To close the cycle and supply the land and its creatures with fresh water, the water evaporates from the sea and is carried across the land by the wind. The connecting force here is again solar energy in the form of heat and the kinetic energy of earlier cosmic events such as the meteorite impact that set the earth in rotation (and incidentally also led to the formation of the moon). Heat leads to the evaporation of water from the sea. The winds that blow the clouds over the land are generated by the interplay between heat and planetary rotation. The winds are therefore an expression of the combined energies at work in our sun, the forces in earlier suns that led to the formation of that meteorite, and the force of gravity that influenced the path of the meteorite so that it could strike the Earth at that time. The next time you feel the wind blowing around your face, think about

the energies and forces that were and are necessary for this to happen. Feeling the wind comes close to being a cosmic experience.

- The connection between water and the human body

The connecting energy is thirst, a physical feeling. It is also an expression of self-preservation. We drink to stay alive. We can last longer without water than without oxygen. Only someone who has been close to dying of thirst can appreciate what an urgent and inescapable feeling thirst is. Without water, death occurs within a few days.

- Carbon atoms combine to form high-energy carbon compounds such as sugar and starch

In this process, which takes place in plants, solar energy is converted into a form that can serve as food for living organisms. The molecule chlorophyll is needed to store solar energy in the form of food. This is a chemical process in which the influence of generative, sustaining and connecting energy is not so easy to recognise. At least not if we look at chlorophyll and the chemical processes involved in starch production in isolation from the whole. The old scientific, compartmentalising approach results in the loss of something essential, namely the overview. When we take a holistic approach, it is not so important how exactly something happens in the smallest detail, but what happens in the whole and what is achieved by the greater whole through this process.
In this example, solar energy is made available to living beings on this planet in a form that is suitable for making life possible at all. Because chlorophyll is necessary for this, the generating energy created this very molecule by radiating

bits of information into the primordial plants so that the information on how to produce this molecule could be embedded in the plants' DNA. The cause of chlorophyll is therefore the primary generative energy, which incidentally also creates all other matter. This stands in contradiction to the theory of evolution, which assumes that the plant simply tries out on its own how to produce something like chlorophyll and by pure chance finds the right DNA formula.

From a holistic perspective, there is no such thing as coincidence. Everything is connected in a meaningful way. A will can therefore be surmised in the greater whole:

**The whole wants energy to be available for life on earth.**

- Connection between food and the body

    The connecting energy is hunger, a physical sensation. This process is also an expression of self-preservation. We eat to stay alive. Only those who have been close to starvation can judge how strong and inescapable hunger can be. Only thirst is stronger.

## On a mental and spiritual level

- Men and women are attracted to each other

    The connecting force is erotic attraction, a special kind of gravity or magnetism, the physical correlate of which is a certain hormonal situation. But that doesn't explain much, because the connecting force behind it has not yet been clearly established. In any case, this force of attraction clearly exists, otherwise humanity would have died out a

33

long time ago or never even come into being. The same applies to the animal kingdom. Sexual attraction operates in the service of species preservation.

- Lovers are attracted to each other

  The active agent here is a spiritual attraction, the primal causes of which are as little understood as the primal causes of gravity. But everyone knows from experience that this kind of spiritual attraction exists. The effects of this force, to which we attribute a loving quality, can be experienced and even measured. Lovers certainly feel the power of attraction very strongly. The hormonal change that is triggered by the presence or even the mere thought of a loved one is actually measurable. Although erotic feelings also play an important role, there is another, additional energy that can be felt when we are in love – a spiritual, loving quality that is the expression of a deeper connection.
  The unifying force at work here is a partial aspect of the all-encompassing love that extends not only to the loved one but also to all aspects of life, essentially to life itself.

- People are connected with the 'blocked' parts of their soul

  This is primarily about parts of the soul that are 'frozen' in a trauma from the personal past. Obviously, the loss of soul parts leads to an unstable psychological situation in which connecting energies are activated that attempt to make the person's soul whole again and to reintegrate the part of the soul left behind.
  There are basically two categories of personal trauma: trauma in a person's current life and trauma in a previous life.

### Personal trauma in current life

The connecting energy manifests itself here as emotional energy. It can take the form of sadness, aggression, fear or physical pain, feelings that are experienced as a disruption to the ideal of a positive attitude towards life that is inherent in every person and serves as an inner compass. The individual begins to suffer. Suffering leads to a search for healing, a search for what is missing. The missing part, the lost part of the soul, can be found under the guidance of a competent therapist. Consciousness plays a decisive role in this process. The individual becomes aware of the traumatic experiences that are part of his or her life. The healing step is to make contact with the part of the soul that became frozen in the trauma and to reintegrate it into the individual's soul. The individual thus becomes complete, whole and healed. The symptoms and illnesses that occur therefore serve the process of becoming whole and healed again.

## The whole aims to integrate
## lost parts of the soul

### Personal trauma in a previous life

Here too, the connecting energy manifests itself as emotional energy, which in some cases can also lead to a manifest physical illness. The symptoms, pain and illnesses can look very similar to childhood trauma. However, the background is different. Trauma in a previous incarnation often involves torture and murder that you have either fallen victim to yourself or, less frequently, that you have committed yourself. As these are usually still energetically active perpetrator-victim fields, the entire field (i.e. all the souls involved) must first be pacified before the part of the soul frozen in the trauma can cross the boundary into the current incarnation and be integrated into the individual's own soul.

Part of this pacification is the creation of two different connections that do not involve the client, but the souls of the people who were involved in the trauma in the previous incarnation.

This pacification of souls cannot be achieved by a human being – neither by the client nor by the healer. It requires the dimension of shamanic healing energies, i.e. healing powers that lie outside the human being and go beyond his or her normal abilities. However, the human being still plays an important role. This is because these healing powers can only take effect when human beings whose training enables them to act as a medium and mediator make themselves available. We humans are needed for our own healing.

On the one hand, the shamanic healing powers bring the perpetrators into contact with the consequences of their actions. On the other hand, the human souls frozen in the trauma are freed from the torpor of the trauma and can continue on their path in peace after all this time, whatever this path may look like.

The shamanic healing energies then bring the part of the soul frozen in the trauma of the previous incarnation to the client.

Under the guidance of the therapist, the conscious integration of this part of the soul can now be performed by the client him- or herself. An enormous release of life energy is regularly experienced.

- People are connected to their clan

The connecting energy here could be called 'bonding love'. The deepest source of bonding love is likewise not yet understood. However, the effects of this connecting force can be experienced. The best-known effects are expressed in family system entanglements, the fact that those born later unconsciously carry the energetic burdens of their ancestors to remind them of those forgotten in the system. In the healing steps that are sought in the family constellation, the forgotten and marginalised are reintegrated into the family. The connecting force expressed in the symptoms and illnesses caused by transgenerational stress is understood in its deeper meaning. Broken connections are restored and thus healed.

## The whole aims to reconnect that which has been separated

Here too, healing goes hand in hand with completion and becoming whole. Consciousness is necessary for this to happen. People must first understand the connections in which they naturally find themselves in their clan before they can agree to them. A separate chapter in this book is devoted to these connections (see chapter 'Trauma in previous generations of the family' starting on page 197).

- People are attracted to their tribe, to their social group

The connecting energy here could be called tribal bonds. This ensured that people formed sufficiently large primary groupings ('hordes') in prehistoric times to ensure the survival of the species.

# The whole wants mankind to survive

The sense of togetherness that this creates leads to enmity with other hordes in the fight for the survival of their own horde when food resources become scarce. This process has also been observed in studies of chimpanzee hordes. Where there is contact with other chimpanzee hordes, it can lead to violent conflict in which chimpanzees kill each other.

For humanity as a whole, this sense of togetherness, which is initially necessary for the survival of the horde, turns into an existential danger when the battle for the better food and other resources leads to hostile nations wiping each other out or even threatening the entire human race with extinction.

But we can also look at the events from a different angle and see the hostility between two tribes or nations as a symptom of a further connecting energy:

- Nations are drawn to each other and clash in wars

The unifying forces here are the power of reconciliation after injustice has been done and the attraction between brothers and sisters who belong together on the level of humanity. Seen in this way, every war can be understood as an attempt by the connecting energy to bring the pre-existing affiliation into the consciousness of those involved and to recognise themselves in the other person. War on a small and large scale can be understood as a disease, a deadly disease, but a disease that ultimately carries the message that we all belong together. Seen from this perspective, war is a sign of the connecting force that causes siblings to clash until, in a leap of consciousness, they recognise the truth of their deep bond. At this point, humanity can be understood as one nation, outside of which there is no nation to fight.

At this point, the connecting force also serves to preserve humanity. Standing on the precipice of annihilation, we might at last realise that we only have a future together. This would actually require a real leap in consciousness, a leap out of the animal instinct of 'us versus them' towards the deep realisation that 'the us includes everyone'. This insight will characterise the people of the future. Something that would bring about real healing on a collective level.

- Human beings are drawn to nature

There is a close connection between mankind and nature. The forces that connect man with nature are expressed in a variety of phenomena. The human body is part of nature. Its substances originate from Mother Earth and return to her after death. Every breath connects man with nature. If nature is poisoned, man is also poisoned. If the earth is exploited, man is also exploited and increasingly robbed of his livelihood. Man's connection with nature is a fact.

When man mentally separates himself from nature – and he can only do this mentally, in other words only in his imagination – then he separates himself from something that belongs to him. The greater whole that man inevitably forms with nature is disrupted. This calls for connecting energies. Because the mental separation from nature is obviously regarded by the greater whole as a mistake that must be corrected. The connecting forces try to restore the lost wholeness in the consciousness of the human being by attracting the attention of the human being with the help of signs such as symptoms, diseases, viral epidemics and natural disasters, similar to a damaged structure in the family system. The dangerous storms and deadly floods caused by climate change and the coronavirus epidemic with its global social and economic consequences are clear examples of this. In order to avert further damage, we are forced to rethink, to recognise the close connection between the fate of the environment and our own fate, and to adapt our actions accordingly. Again, awareness is the most important factor. We must first recognise our connections with nature in order to consent to them and let our actions be guided by this realisation.

## The whole wants awareness

The full impact of the negative effects of environmental destruction on human health is still far from being recognised. When someone dies in flooding caused by climate change, the link to environmental damage is clear. If someone develops a cancerous tumour because they have eaten radioactively contaminated fish from the Pacific, it may take years or decades before the link is scientifically proven. We cannot wait until a sufficiently large number of individual cases are investigated to prove that our mental separation from nature – our selfish arrogance, which makes us believe that we are superior to nature – is the underlying cause of so many diseases and relationship problems.

The time for awareness is today. We now need to see the big picture and trust in our intuitive perceptive ability which opens our eyes to the obvious. We need a collective elevation of consciousness that makes reality clear to us. Only then will we still have a chance as humanity on this planet. Only then can the tide turn.

### Energies that separate

It may seem to be only of philosophical interest at this point, but to grasp the whole, we need to answer the question of what the separating energies look like. For it is obvious that they must exist. Otherwise there would be no need for connecting energies. So, what are the energies that cause the actual or mental separation of parts of a whole and thus create a tension that needs to be resolved by connecting energies?

Let's start again with one of the most obvious connecting energies, namely gravity:

In order for gravity to have an effect, the constituent parts of matter must first be spatially separated from one another. At the same time as matter is created, space must also be stretched out. Without space, all matter would be compressed into an unimaginably small point. The effects of gravity would not be recognisable there, because without space there can be no movement. One could also say that, in this state, gravity has exerted its maximum effect because it has compressed all matter into a tiny point. But it could also be that matter does not exist at all without space in between. In other words, matter and the space in between would have been created simultaneously by the primary energy. Matter would therefore have been created by a separating, space-creating energy. We would have identified the creating energy as the separating agent, at least on this level. The separating energy is therefore necessary so that the basis for life can be created.

### The whole needs separation as a prerequisite for life

At the level of hydrogen atoms, we can take this idea further and assume that the primary energy has created the hydrogen atoms in a separate and therefore highly energised form. Each hydrogen atom exists initially for itself. Only through this initial situation can the sun provide its energy in the evenly dispensed form that we need for life. Separation is necessary to create the tension that introduces movement into living processes.

## Separation makes life possible

After the energy for life has been made available in a compatible form, and after other material prerequisites for life have been created (e.g. the existence of a suitable planet and organic substances such as chlorophyll), the interplay of separating and connecting energies begins in order to keep life in action.

The human organism must connect with oxygen, for which the breathing reflex is required; it must supply itself with water, for which the sensation of thirst is required; and it must supply itself with food, for which the sensation of hunger is required. In addition to all these connecting energies, there is also the separating energy. The carbon dioxide produced by internal combustion must leave the body through exhalation, the water must leave the body through the urinary system, laden with many metabolic waste products. The food leaves the body in a modified form through the intestines or bound to oxygen as carbon dioxide. The energy stored in the food leaves the body in the form of action energy and body heat.

## Life means the alternation of separation and connection

On the mental-spiritual level, the separating energies that require a connecting movement to balance them out are somewhat different. Let us first look at the separation of relationships based on love. The separating agent in loving relationships could be called 'fate' or 'destiny'. It is primarily about premature separations that take place at a time when the arc of the relationship has not yet been completed. Examples of this type of fate are death through illness, natural disasters, accidents, murder, suicide or death on the battlefield. Separations caused by flight from danger or due to intolerable situations such as jealousy and violence also fall into this category. Another type of fate is the disruption or destruction of a romantic relationship due to the stress experienced by one or both partners arising from unresolved traumas in childhood or in earlier generations of the family.

An unresolved trauma in a previous life can also trigger a separation in the current life, especially if the previous incarnation was shared with the same partner. When two people meet for the first time and fall in love, many assume that they have never met before, and that therefore no separating force was ever necessary to trigger this kind of attractional bonding force. However, it may be that the lovers know each other from one or more previous lives, were separated prematurely and therefore meet again in this life in order to fulfil this love, to continue and complete the arc of love.

The influences of previous incarnations on the psyche are still little researched, at least in Western science. It could be that many or perhaps even all people who meet in this life, either privately or professionally, were already connected to each other in previous lives. The fact that there are many more people living on earth at the moment than in the past does not in principle argue against this, because it is possible that people have incarnated on other planets in the vastness of the universe and that the pool of souls that can be drawn from is therefore infinite.

Further examples of separating fate:

- Separation of parents and child due to early death of a parent or child

- Separation of a child from its father or mother after the parents have separated

- Separation from siblings due to early death

- Separation of a person from their ideal, inherent path in life and thus making their destiny or vocation impossible because of internal restrictive thought patterns, because of blocking feelings such as fear or unconscious solidarity with one's family of origin or social class

But what is the separating energy that triggers these kinds of blows of fate? Is there such a thing as a primary separating energy of fate? Does the separating fate act in the service of life, in the same way as the separating, space-creating primary energy?

Or is divisive fate triggered by negative, murderous energies that are fundamentally hostile to life?

In family and symptom constellations, we repeatedly encounter a negative, destructive energy that holds some perpetrators, especially mass murderers, in its thrall. Where this deeply negative, all-life-destroying energy comes from and what purpose it serves in the world remains a mystery. What is certain is that it is responsible for many traumatic separations in the history of mankind.

Ultimately, divisive fate is an inevitable part of life. Life happens in the interplay of separation and connection. But even if separation creates the space in which a new or renewed connection can take place, it is always the (re)connection that is experienced in a pleasurable and redeeming way. Connection leads to healing, while separation is often associated with pain and suffering. As human beings, we move and operate within this field of tension.

The meaning behind this is a mystery that mankind has been trying to decipher since the very beginning of civilisation. It must somehow lie in the generative and sustaining energies, in other words in the big picture. For if there is to be a meaning, then it lies in the very beginnings. In this case, the greater whole has something to do with life, has an intention, a direction. We always need to keep the greater whole in mind in this book when we look at the smaller parts. Because only when we look at the greater whole do our insights appear in a new light. Perhaps this will give us an idea of what the greater whole actually intends to do with us when it pushes us into separation, in order to then provide us with the healing powers and the necessary awareness that will in turn bring us connection and healing.

If there is an intention of the greater whole, there must be an energy at the helm. The fact that these controlling energies actually exist can be seen in the material, biological processes.

### Energies that regulate or control

The regulating or controlling energies are a further type of energy which, in order to grasp them better, we can initially regard as something independent. These energies must exist. Because it is wrong to assume that the matter generated by the primary energy and sustained in every millisecond is capable of regulating and controlling itself.

The clearest example of this can be found in embryonic development. The stem cells, which are formed by identical division of the fertilised egg cell, are in urgent need of the information as to which cell type they should develop into. Should they become liver cells, blood cells, bone cells, muscle cells or rather nerve cells? At DNA level, no gene has been found that could provide this information, because all cells have identical DNA. The information impulse must come from outside, from an energetic information field.

So there are controlling energies that are important and necessary for embryonic development, for the formation of human life. This leads us to believe that other – perhaps even all – bodily processes also benefit from these controlling energies and are indeed completely dependent on them.

We are familiar with many control circuits at a physical level, e.g. the regulation of the hormonal situation. It is known that the pituitary gland is the controlling organ at this level. However, the pituitary gland – this small pineal gland in the centre of the brain – is itself a recipient of commands and is only a relay station for the transmission of information. The actual control centre lies on an energetic level outside the body. An exact location is not going to be found. This is because the energetic control centre, which controls the hormonal situation of every human being, is everywhere and nowhere. It is connected to the greater whole by invisible connections, just like everything else. The greater whole controls. The regulating and controlling energies are only the extended arm of the greater whole, which radiates into everything. It is also connected to a person's life path. Whatever is behind those processes, it is not a coincidence.

The greater whole has a plan.

## Energy and connection

What exactly is connection? When two people are connected, that seems obvious to us. There is an exchange of energy, information and emotions.

But when connection becomes a state of being in which an individual, like all matter, is ultimately just energy and connection, then a dimension opens up that puts our understanding to the test. Because then connection is not something between two parts or two people, but also something within a part, even the very essence of its being. At this point, the separated part that is so important to our mind dissolves and connects with the whole. Connection is thus the perceptible expression of the existence of wholeness.

The human being is therefore also an expression of wholeness. The following section will focus on the human being. What is the human being's position in all these energetic structures, in all these connecting energies? Perhaps we will even get to the bottom of the big question of what the human being actually is.

We already know that the human being is an integral energetic entity of a large, energetic whole. The energetic entity that is the human being does not cease to exist when the body is discarded at death. That which lives on, we call the soul. As this term is used frequently in the following, I would like to define how I use it in this book.

## The term 'soul'

For the purpose of this book, it is best to detach the term soul from all religious concepts. It is something quite normal – you are a soul, I am a soul and we have our body for a while. When we discard this body at death, we continue to exist as a soul. All feelings and even inner attitudes remain with the soul, wherever it goes.

I do not know the path that a soul has to take after the death of the body. Finding out more about this path would be interesting from a philosophical point of view, but it is not necessary for the successful practice of energy medicine. I know very well from decades of working with symptom constellations that the human being continues to exist as a soul and takes all emotions with him or her. Otherwise it would not be possible to recognise the emotional state of the deceased in a constellation. This is because, in constellations, we never look into the past but always into the present moment, into the current state of mind of living and dead people. It may be the imprint of the past in the present emotional world of the person concerned. But it is always the present state of mind of a soul that we look at in a constellation, whether it still has a body or not.

If you know this, you can also understand that the mental states of the living and the dead can change while we work with them in a healing way today. Otherwise we would not be able to understand the healing effects that we regularly see after constellations and shamanic healings. Because what happened yesterday or fifty or a hundred years ago cannot be changed.

There is no separation of soul and body during life. They are united during this time. What happens to the body also happens to the soul and what happens to the soul also happens to the body.

## Chapter 2: The human energy field

Human beings exist in an energy field that completely surrounds them as an aura, but which also permeates every single cell of the body. This energy field contains various energy qualities, some of which are supportive and beneficial, while others are harmful and pathogenic. You can imagine this energy field as an aura that permeates the body, an energy cloud in which there are different coloured areas – coloured clouds that sometimes flow together, overlap or separate off from each other. Emotional qualities sit and vibrate in this energy field. For example, you can imagine anger and aggression as a deep red mist, sadness and depression as black or dark, fear and panic as blue, despair as purple, peaceful relaxation as green, joy as light yellow and love as pink. The human energy field is not static, but more or less in motion. Some areas swirl strongly, others are stuck and locked in place.

It is interesting to note that this energy field does not end with a hard boundary somewhere a metre or two away from the body, but is instead connected to the energy fields of other people, including the deceased, along fine or sometimes strong energetic pathways. There are also connections to the energy fields of plants, animals, the energy field of the earth and therefore also to the cosmic energies of the universe. There are also connections to those parts of the human soul that were left behind in a past trauma. You can also imagine these diverse connections as oscillating radiations through which energy flows in and out.

Energy medicine is particularly interested in disruptive and pathogenic energies. Where do they come from and to which nearby or distant energy fields are they connected?

In my work as a doctor and system constellator, four main areas have crystallised as sources of disruptive energies:

1. Trauma that we have experienced in our own current life, e.g. in childhood or adolescence

2. Trauma that we have experienced in a previous incarnation

3. Transgenerational trauma experienced by a family member of the same generation (siblings) or a previous generation (parents, grandparents etc) or inflicted by that family member on other people

4. Loss trauma in the family of which you are the founder (present family). This applies to current or former lovers and spouses and all your own children, including miscarried, aborted or deceased children.

What all these areas have in common is that the stressful energies are the result of unresolved traumas in the past. It is therefore important to understand what trauma is and how unresolved trauma affects the human energy field and therefore mental and physical health. Trauma is the key concept in understanding how to use energy medicine for healing purposes.

**Trauma**

The word 'trauma' comes from the Greek and broadly means 'injury'.

Injuries occur at all levels of human existence. Physical injuries caused by an accident are referred to as traumas, as are psychological injuries. Often both body and soul are affected by an injury.

Trauma in the classic sense is a one-off or repeated event that is so threatening and incisive that it leads to a feeling of helplessness and defenceless abandonment. The trauma violates physical or mental integrity or threatens life.

In the case of **personal trauma**, the traumatic event only affects one person, at least superficially. Examples include a serious accident, kidnapping, torture, rape, sexual abuse, maltreatment or violent or forced separation.

**Collective trauma** by definition affects many people, also fulfils the criterion of an extraordinary threat and causes deep despair in almost everyone, e.g. natural disasters or man-made, catastrophic circumstances such as combat operations, war, genocide, displacement, flight, terrorism or witnessing the violent death of other people.

Trauma is part of life. We cannot avoid traumatic events. People have experienced them throughout history.

You may have been traumatised in a previous incarnation. If you have suffered a violent death in a previous life, it is possible that your soul has not yet come to terms with this trauma and is still carrying this burden as energy into the new life.

Trauma can already occur in the womb in an individual's current life. A child senses when the mother is sad because, for example, there has been a separation or some other tragic circumstance has arisen. If a twin dies during pregnancy, this is also a trauma for the surviving child.

Birth can also be traumatic or the child can experience separation trauma in the first few days or years if it is taken away from its mother after birth (just a few minutes are enough) or if it has to be admitted to hospital later due to illness and the parents have to leave the child there alone, as was common in the past. Or a child experiences serious accidents, the early death of a parent or sibling. Or a person, as an adult, becomes a victim of one of the major collective traumas mentioned above such as war or terrorism.

In the case of **transgenerational trauma,** you do not experience the trauma yourself. It happened to a family member of a previous generation, e.g. parents, grandparents or great-grandparents. Or it was inflicted on other people by a family member.

Nevertheless, descendants suffer from the consequences of unresolved trauma, which are passed on from generation to generation via epigenetic mechanisms in the unconscious energy field of the family.

## Basic mechanisms in the trauma process

To understand what happens in a person's energy fields as a result of trauma, we first look at the basic psychological and physical mechanisms that are triggered by trauma.

### Physical and emotional shutdown

In acutely threatening situations (e.g. when a lion attacks), all physical and emotional channels of perception immediately shut down. This is an automatic, physiological reaction that is unavoidable and that we cannot influence with willpower. This is a feature we have in common with animals.

In this state, you no longer feel any pain or fear. Inwardly and outwardly frozen, you no longer need to suffer the deadly bite or the blow from the lion's paw. We are spared this by nature. In this respect, shutdown makes sense.

However, it is also possible that the emotional shutdown only blocks the feelings that occur from this point onwards. In such cases, however, the feelings of the moment in which the shutdown begins – the pain, suffering and horror – continue to be experienced over and over again. Time stands still and no longer plays a role, regardless of whether years, decades or centuries pass. The affected soul continues to experience the traumatic situation as if in an endless loop. I refer to such very common cases as 'trauma freeze'.

If the victim survives the threatening situation, it is possible that a part of his or her soul does not realise that it has been saved and perceives itself as still being in the life-threatening situation. Because this happens in the subconscious, the survivor is unaware of it and simply tries to go on living as if nothing significant had happened. The shut-down part of the soul left behind in the dangerous situation (which always has a physical equivalent somewhere in the body) can still be reactivated years and decades later in situations that are only remotely reminiscent of the trauma situation at the time. An adult can then suddenly feel like a small child in a life-threatening situation, feeling panic, fear, anger or the urge to flee from an intimate situation as if under duress. Neither the persons affected nor those around them understand what is happening, what has suddenly snapped. Heartache, abdominal pain, coughing, allergies, itching, nausea or emotional reactions such as acute sadness or sudden lethargy and tiredness can also be signs of such an inner reactivation of a traumatised part of the soul.

All of these symptoms, which are summarised under the technical term 'post-traumatic stress disorder' (PTSD), are the consequences of unresolved trauma.

### Frozen feelings in non-fatal trauma

In the case of non-lethal trauma, a part of the soul or a 'soul quality' can freeze. However, the emotional energy frozen by the trauma does not disappear by blocking the channels of perception. The feelings are still there; they are just repressed into the unconscious and thus permanently enter into the energy field of the person affected. The most important emotional qualities here are fear, pain and rage, which can be reactivated later in life in situations similar to those described above.

### Frozen feelings in fatal trauma

In the event of a violent death, the entire soul can become frozen in the trauma situation. In the trauma freeze, this soul then either no longer perceives death at all, continues to feel itself in the trauma situation or remains dully and numbly attached to the body in death. In both cases, it is not possible for the affected soul to follow the path that a soul should take after the death of the body. This makes any further development impossible. The feelings that, in this case, pass into the unconscious energy field of this soul and can remain there for decades or even centuries are, in addition to fear, pain and anger, above all hopelessness, despair and sadness about the impossible path into the light.

This energetic stagnation is a burden for the affected soul, but also leads to lasting stress in later generations of both the victim's family and that of the perpetrator. This is because all the emotional qualities described above pass from the energy field of the murdered person to the energy fields of both the victim's and the perpetrator's family, where they can spread to the children and grandchildren in later generations.

For the soul of the perpetrator who murders someone or even only indirectly contributes to the murder of other people, the deed also represents a trauma. Even if he or she rejects this fact on a conscious level, his or her soul still suffers from having committed the crime. A part of the perpetrator's soul can also freeze in the act, so that the murder is not over and done with on the energy level for the murderer's soul either, but still takes place again and again. The murderous aggression of the perpetrator and also the deep grief of a part of the perpetrator's soul caused by the deed then lies in the energy field of the murderer for decades or sometimes centuries and burdens the energy fields of the coming generations of the family of the perpetrator and the victim. This results in aggression flaring up over generations, which can lead to auto-aggressive diseases or fatal accidents, but also to new acts of violence such as repeating murders or suicides.

Bert Hellinger, the founder of family constellations, coined the term 'systemic entanglement' to describe these processes.

# How to avoid permanent trauma stress

The negative consequences (PTSD) after a personal experience of trauma and the intergenerational burden after a trauma suffered by a family member are avoidable. This is because not every traumatic event necessarily leads to stressful after-effects. It depends on how the affected persons and those around them deal with it.

An optimal, healthy way of dealing with trauma involves recognising that the event is a trauma and therefore requires a special approach. The traumatised persons need help and understanding from those around them. The community has an important role to play: in the ideal case, people show solidarity, they talk repeatedly about the event. And, above all, the feelings that are triggered by a trauma as a healthy reaction must be allowed to show themselves, to be given space. Horror, grief and anger must be allowed to express themselves. Healthy trauma processing takes time and requires a knowledgeable environment and skilled helpers. The traumatised persons should have the feeling that they are not being left alone with what has happened and their reactions. They need time and an accepting, supportive environment so that they can move on from the traumatic experience into a life after the trauma, with their soul intact.

If this is successful, the trauma is resolved and has no burdening consequences. However, if it does not succeed or is not attempted at all, we speak of 'unresolved trauma', which can be expected to have stressful consequences later on.

Characteristics of a problematic response to trauma are indifference, looking away, playing down, concealing, wanting to forget or active suppression of adequate emotional reactions by other people in the victim's surroundings. A healthy approach to trauma will attempt to avoid these mistakes, to provide support and guidance and, in addition, to actively care for the closed-down part of the soul and to promote its reopening and reintegration into the overall personality as soon as possible after the trauma.

Because many personal traumas, as well as major collective traumas such as war, genocide and expulsion, could not be dealt with in this way, we live in a society in which we encounter the unconscious consequences of unresolved trauma at every turn. Whether we like it or not, we have to deal with it personally and as a society every day. But we often don't realise it.

The greatest realisation and the basis for any further understanding of the phenomenon of trauma is the fact that an unresolved trauma shows a strong, often irresistible urge to repeat itself. Accidents, illnesses or other blows of fate are repeated over generations. Wars keep breaking out. Political oppression keeps being perpetrated.

In order to break the cycle of repetition, it is necessary to track down and heal the traumas of the past, both on a personal and collective level. This is precisely what is now possible with energy medicine. A new era is dawning.

### How stresses in the human energy field lead to physical and mental symptoms and illnesses

The energies in an individual's energy field vary in their nature. They can be positive or negative, i.e. beneficial to life and health or detrimental, causing disorders such as illness and emotional stress.

The way in which an energy relates to the quality of the connection is of paramount importance. Remember! Matter is energy and connection. The human being is also energy and connection. That is why the body is nothing else and can be nothing else but energy and connection. Energy is force, a force that seeks to have an effect, but which can only have an effect if it is connected to other areas of energy.

An ideal connection that is healthy for the body and soul is one that flows freely. Free-flowing energy is health, blocked energy leads to illness. In order to understand what happens when energy is blocked, we must assume the existence of a blocking energy. Because nothing happens without a reason. There is always an energy-based cause for a process. There is always an energy involved, in this case a blocking energy.

What can this blocking energy be, and where does it come from?

## Feelings

This is where feelings play a decisive role. Because feelings are carried by energy. In the human energy field, there are different emotional energies of varying intensity. Firstly, a list of the main emotional qualities:

- Love
- Joy
- Grief and depression
- Anger and aggression
- Fear
- Pain
- Despair
- Shame
- Feeling of guilt
- Feeling of revenge
- Feeling of arrogance
- Feeling of disappointment
- Feeling of isolation

## Love

Love is the primary feeling. Love is an expression of existing connections. Through the feeling of love, the connection to the object of affection is brought to consciousness, revered and confirmed in its importance. This object of affection can be oneself, another person, an activity, a thing, nature or even the entire universe.

Apparently, there is an ideal, paradisiacal state of being in which you know you are connected to everything through the power of love. In this state, nothing is missing. You are filled with love, contentment and joy. Consciousness plays the decisive role here.

Connectedness and love, in which one feels the joy of connection, is the basis of our being – a fact of life in general. That is why love cannot be driven away, but only concealed, suffocated or denied. Nevertheless, it continues to exist at its core.

## Joy

Joy arises when love is allowed to be and connections are able to flow freely. Joy carries a special energy that clearly shows us that something is all right now or will be soon. In this context, 'all right' means that the connections flow freely and are experienced in a lively way. You are happy about having received a hug, a look, a word; you may even be able to sense when a loved one is thinking of you. You are happy to receive a gift, a letter or nowadays a WhatsApp message or a Like on Facebook.

We are joyful about food that provides us with good nourishment and thus connects us with nature. We are joyful that we are needed. We are also joyful about professional success, which shows that the community is happy to accept what we provide as a service or good.

We enjoy movement that connects us with our body. The feeling of joy can make us realise that we are also connected to our body through love. It simply triggers joy when we give the body what it needs to feel good.

We are happy about beauty that we encounter – a beautiful person, a mountain, a tree, a flower, a poem, a painting or the décor of a room. Here, too, it is the joy of an inner resonance, a sublime connection that we feel with beauty.

# Grief

Grief is a primordial feeling. Grief always has a cause, a reason. It never comes from nothing. The reason is the loss of a loved one or a homeland, a place, sometimes even a physical object.

Like any emotion, grief must be able to flow if it is to fulfil its deeper meaning. It announces a connection that we are in, sometimes without realising it. The strength of the grief reflects the strength of the connection and thus also the strength of the love that we have felt or still feel for a person.

Consequently, grief does not contradict love, it does not conceal or extinguish it, but is instead an expression of it. Flowing tears of grief are also free-flowing love.

The connection to another person, a community or even a landscape is sometimes much deeper than we realised before the loss. When the loss occurs, it is the mourning that makes us realise the depth of the connection. This realisation puts something right. Because when we know the depth of a connection, we can honour and fully accept it. This makes us more complete, healthier, happier; even though it comes to us in and through a state of grief. Mourning honours the connection, honours the love.

If you allow grief to take its full course, you sometimes receive a gift in its depths, namely the realisation that the connection may continue to exist. It allows you to remain emotionally connected to the loved one you have just lost through separation or death. This realisation soothes and fills you with joy.

But grief also hurts. The pain can sometimes seem almost unbearable. But if you bear it, it can subside again after a while. Grief takes time. It comes in waves, whereby the waves get smaller over time, provided you allow the grief to flow freely.

If there are difficulties because an individual is unable to grieve or the grief does not subside over time, it may be that there are blockages in the unconscious energy field of the mourner from earlier traumas of loss. In this case, the old trauma must first be located and released. Only then can the current grief flow and attain its goal of revealing love.

### Anger and aggression

Anger always has a cause. As a rule, the triggering moment is an injury or an infringement of one's personal space, a physical attack, an insult or an injustice. The feeling of anger builds up aggression.

Aggression is not entirely negative, but essentially value-neutral. The word can be traced back to the Latin 'aggredere', which means 'to advance' or 'to move forward'. We have to move forward in life, otherwise there would be no development.

### Positive aggression

Here we find many reactions that we also know from the animal kingdom and that fulfil important functions both there and in human communities. They serve self-preservation and species conservation, but also the preservation and development of an existing community (family, horde, society, state).

Positive aggression is a part of life energy. We can imagine that the great life energy that is in all living things flows into positive aggression in one of its arms.

Here too, as in physics, the law of conservation of energy applies. This states that energy cannot disappear without a trace; it can only change into another form.

Like any other life energy, positive aggression must be able to flow and exert an effect. If it cannot do this because it is blocked for whatever reason, it will have a destructive effect in the place where it has arisen, in a person or collectively in a society. The question in the face of a disturbance or destruction is therefore always: Is it a case of blocked positive aggression that has not yet reached its destination, or is it a case of negative, fundamentally destructive aggression?

**Areas in which we encounter positive aggression:**

**Self-preservation:**
**Defensive aggression** builds up during an attack. You defend yourself or your family or horde. This is quite natural and necessary to ensure survival.

The basics of life, resources such as water, food, supplies, the cave, the fire pit and possessions are also defended.

**Species conservation:**
After self-preservation, the next priority in nature is preservation of the species. The sex drive leads to a special kind of forward step. You have to venture forth from your cosy fireside and visit the neighbouring cave to find a suitable sexual partner.

The very act of showing yourself represents a form of aggression. You have left the dark corner of the cave, straightened up and made yourself visible. This is healthy and life affirming. Anyone who finds this act of self-manifestation difficult will sooner or later experience this as a restriction. Because people want to be visible. They have the urge to play their part in preserving the species. Even the attempt brings a certain degree of fulfilment. Those who withdraw from the process suffer the consequences.

**Preservation of society:**
Next, the tribe must be preserved. Without the tribe, survival in the wilderness was often not possible. This includes the **struggle for leadership positions**. The best and strongest are the ones who should lead, so that society has the best chance of surviving and developing.

61

In some societies, there is a feeling that the best and most capable are not leading, thereby indicating that the battle for leadership positions has not been waged or has in some way been frustrated. This does not mean that the healthy aggression that is needed here is not present. It is perhaps blocked, because those against whom the aggression should be directed are not visible: those who are actually in power hide behind a wall of silence and control the politicians in the spotlight like puppets. If one of their puppets is lost, it is no big deal. The puppet can be replaced. The people pulling the strings retain power. But if the common good of society is taken as the yardstick, they are not necessarily the best and most capable.

The collective unconscious cannot be fooled. The positive aggression that wants the best and most capable to lead remains present and eventually becomes mobilised. When it is blocked, there are tendencies towards auto-aggression in society, conflicts between ethnic groups and an increased level of aggression in society as a whole. Or the opposite happens, a collective depression that is unconsciously intended to protect against destructive outbreaks of violence in the community.

These phenomena have been observed in many societies during the coronavirus pandemic. The next few years will also provide an opportunity to study collective phenomena of this kind. This is because positive aggression, which seeks to bring the most capable into leadership positions, will not disappear. It is a primordial elementary component of human societies. The people living under a dictatorship, regardless of political spectrum, will eventually rise up. It is only a question of time.

The **fight for freedom** of each individual or entire population groups also falls under this category. The aggression that facilitates this struggle is also primordial. If freedom of movement is constrained, people will fight against the restriction or move on ('aggredere' in the sense of the Latin verb) and look for a living space in which such a restriction does not exist.

The **fight for justice** also serves to secure the existence of the community. Systematic injustice leads to insecurity and manifestations of disintegration.

The **struggle for fair distribution** of goods, of what is hunted and harvested, also belongs in the category of 'positive aggression'. The fact that a fair distribution of goods has not yet been achieved in many parts of the world does not mean that this type of aggression does not exist. It also exists and has an effect. As it is often blocked, it has mainly negative effects. It disrupts society and can even destroy it.

### Special case: Revenge aggression

When your own family, your own people are attacked, defensive aggression arises. If it is unsuccessful because you are too weak or have become trapped or are afraid to intervene so as not to endanger your own life, or because you arrive on the scene too late, then defensive aggression turns into revenge aggression.

However, it is important to distinguish between two types of revenge aggression:

- Primary revenge aggression directed at the actual perpetrators of an assault
- Secondary revenge aggression directed at the descendants or the ethnic group or people of the perpetrators

In early societies, the primary aggression of revenge was directed at the perpetrators. Revenge was enacted personally and the murderer was also murdered by the avenger. Although this initially brought quick compensation, it had the disadvantage that one became a perpetrator oneself and in turn attracted revenge, despite being 'only' a just avenger.

In civilised societies, primary revenge aggression is satisfied by disempowering and disarming the perpetrators and punishing them through an established judicial system. This type of revenge aggression can be appeased and pacified by righteous punishment, because it has already been carried out in this case.

Secondary revenge aggression is directed at innocent people who have no personal involvement in the original offence, e.g. descendants or members of the murderer's ethnic group. This is not a just punishment here, because the targets are innocent. Those who take revenge on innocent people also become perpetrators themselves.

The idea that peace can be found by taking revenge on the descendants of the perpetrators or the members of their ethnic group or nation is illusory. The result is not peace, but a revenge-driven cascade of murders and wars in which the roles of perpetrator and victim are often exchanged. A 'family of victims' becomes a 'family of perpetrators', a 'nation of victims' becomes a 'nation of perpetrators'. These repetitions of trauma and war can last for decades in families and, at the collective level of nations, for many centuries or even millennia.

Primary revenge aggression in its civilised form brings about peace, because it creates a real balance that is effective in the soul. Secondary revenge aggression creates conflict and war through an endless cascade of war and suffering fuelled by blind revenge.

The difference is also visible in the effects of blocked aggression. If the primary aggression of revenge is blocked, the aggression of revenge is circling around in ourselves and our own descendants. It leads to self-harm via auto-aggressive diseases and even depression-induced suicide.

If the secondary aggression of revenge is blocked and controlled, it leads to peace for us and our descendants. The vicious circle of the vendetta is interrupted.

## The negative aggression of the perpetrator

In addition to positive aggression, which protects and develops life, there is also negative aggression, which destroys life and makes social progress impossible.

This includes the aggression of perpetrators, i.e. people who harm or murder innocent people. Negative aggression also has an origin and, if it has taken hold in the energy field of a person or a group of people, can continue to come and go in waves over generations or collectively over centuries, perhaps lying dormant in the unconscious for a while, only to suddenly resurface. As a result, an old trauma is often repeated in a new and later time.

Philosophers around the world have long pondered the question of where the origin of negative aggression really lies. However, there is still no definitive answer to this question. Has negative aggression – negativity per se – always been rooted in man himself or was there a paradisiacal time when this type of aggression had not yet entered the world and peace prevailed? In which case, the next question is, of course, who or what brought negative aggression into the world.

I can't give a definitive answer to this question either. However, work on constellations has contributed something interesting, perhaps even groundbreaking, to our understanding of this area. Above all, working as a medium for the shamanic healing powers of Healing Voices has opened my eyes to the nature of negative aggression.

It seems that there really is a negative force in the universe that is able to possess people, to take over the command centre in the area of the brain that controls willpower and to operate through the actions of these people. Sometimes the energy field of mass murderers has shown the energy of something absolutely negative, something absolutely evil, which, equipped with a high level of aggression, is intent only on destroying everything living and beautiful.

Why some people allow themselves to be affected by negative energy and others do not is still a mystery. Perhaps future research will shed more light on this area. The fact is, however, that perpetrators can be affected by this negative energy, some more than others.

This is most evident in the healing movements triggered by the shamanic healing forces in the constellations of war crimes. The souls of the perpetrators who have entered into too close a relationship with the negative forces must leave the system with these forces. They are disempowered and their energy is destroyed. In this way, a delayed form of justice is meted out and order is restored. It is only then that healing of the victims becomes possible. The descendants are also liberated from the energy of the perpetrators.

The souls of the perpetrators who have not entered into such an intimate relationship with the negative forces can be released from these negative forces by shamanic healing powers. In these cases, only the negative energies are destroyed and leave the system, while the perpetrator remains in the system. In this case, however, the perpetrator is transformed, suddenly becomes human again (as if he had previously been inhuman), feels his heart again, becomes compassionate towards the victims, suddenly sees what he has done, breaks down in remorse in front of the victims and weeps bitterly over his actions. This can take a very long time. The process of remorse can continue for weeks and months after a shamanic healing. But for the souls of these perpetrators, this is obviously the only way forward. The descendants do not have to worry about this. In this case, they are also liberated from the energy of the offender and can go their own way (more on this in the chapter 'Healing Voices' starting on page 116).

Negative aggression is found in war criminals, mass murderers, torturers, often also in individual perpetrators and, in various forms, in all perpetrators involved in the numerous trauma and war repetitions that follow an original trauma over the decades and centuries.

Sometimes, negative aggression is also found in people who acquire property unlawfully and subsequently defend this property as if they had a genuine right to it. Negative aggression can also be found in people who hoard power and possessions, albeit covertly. This type of aggression is not linked to life energy, but leads to the destruction of societies and prosperity. It is a threat to peace.

## Fear

Fear is initially a sensible emotional response to danger. Fear activates defence and protective reactions that protect life and health. Fear manifests itself equally in emotions and body reactions.

Think, for example, of the physical reaction that is automatically triggered by a precipice in the mountains as soon as you get too close to it. This reaction can be felt in the abdomen in a matter of seconds. Your attention is immediately focused on the ground, your sense of balance is mobilised and your arms make compensatory balancing movements to prevent a fall. You are afraid to get any closer to the cliff edge and look for safe ground.

If you spend the night in a cave and suddenly hear the roaring of a lion, fear immediately sets in. You either try to get to safety, or freeze so as not to give away your own presence or prepare for a fight by reaching for your weapon. Your heart beats faster, your blood pressure rises and your senses become more acute.

Without the capacity to feel fear, our ancestors would not have survived and we would not exist today. The fear response, the ability to sense danger, is deeply primordial. Normally and ideally, this type of fear disappears once the danger has been overcome. We return to a healthy basic state of relaxation, like a gazelle that escapes from a lion, shakes itself off briefly and then continues to graze calmly.

However, in the case of a traumatic event so overwhelming that it forces its way through our mental and physical defences, the fear may become frozen in a part of the soul, remain in the unconscious as 'trembling' energy and harden into an emotional time bomb. Even decades later, this fear can be reactivated by an event reminiscent of the trauma at the time and trigger all the symptoms of a post-traumatic stress reaction, e.g. a panic attack or physical pain.

In this case, fear has lost all its protective function and disrupts life. It may accompany an individual through life like a form of background noise. The individual then becomes anxious, does not have the confidence to carry out certain activities and gets a tight feeling in lifts, in crowds, when driving, in exam situations, when flying or in intimate situations. As if under duress, he or she feels compelled to flee the situation. Life becomes restricted. The space which the individual inhabits becomes small and cramped.

Sometimes, however, the fear is buried so deeply in the unconscious that the individual does not notice it in everyday life. It can erupt all the more vehemently in a full-blown panic attack when something happens that is reminiscent of the original trauma.

These phenomena also occur at the collective level of society. In every society there is an unconscious domain in which the potential for fear is encapsulated. It has arisen in collective, unresolved traumas of the past.

In a situation that is even remotely reminiscent of the original trauma, people suddenly become inexplicably afraid, even though the current situation does not explain the extent of the fear. This phenomenon was readily observable during the coronavirus crisis. The devastating pandemics of the past, such as the plague or the Spanish flu of 1918-1920, can be assumed to be the original trauma. During the coronavirus outbreak, the potential for fear, which had been dormant in the collective unconscious for decades or centuries, erupted vehemently and sometimes intensified the anxiety of the present to the point of grotesqueness.

When an individual is at the mercy of unconscious fear, he or she freezes inwardly and becomes incapable of level-headed behaviour. If this happens to many people at the same time, the whole of society freezes and is deprived of its healthy mental agility. In a state of collective anxiety neurosis, society becomes vulnerable to political manipulation. Collective fear is therefore often misused as an instrument of political power, whipped up by targeted propaganda, and becomes entrenched in the state of mind of the population as a chronic weakening. For just as a panic attack robs an individual of his or her ability to act and of cool-headed deliberation, a population filled with fear is also incapable of acting, can no longer think coolly and logically and follows the instructions of authority uncritically and with trembling limbs, even feeling grateful for any instruction that promises security. The aggression behind every fear can then be channelled at will by politicians, typically at those sections of the population who, for whatever reason, refuse to be intimidated.

Ultimately, though, no one is really free from collective fear.

For a society to become immune to political manipulation, the collective traumas from long ago such as the plague or the Spanish flu would have to be healed. This is possible today through collective system constellations in combination with shamanic healing powers.

The same phenomenon can be seen in armed conflict such as the current war in Ukraine. The fear of war is also spreading in countries that are not presently at risk. This is because the traumas of the First and Second World Wars are still deeply embedded in the unconscious of the nations involved. These fears can easily be fuelled by targeted propaganda. Populations can be manipulated and readily accept political decisions that they would never have countenanced just a few weeks before. What matters to them is that these measures serve national security.

However, the opposite is the case: by fuelling fears that lie dormant in the unconscious from earlier wars, the repetition of the trauma in the form of a new war on old terrain becomes more likely. The danger of war increases!

Most people do not realise that the fear they feel is perhaps only the fear felt by their ancestors who lived through those earlier wars. They do not realise that the fear is passed on from generation to generation in the energy field of the family or the nation. This ignorance impinges on the freedom of the descendants and the current society and significantly hinders their development and progress.

The solution is firstly knowledge of how everything is connected over time and secondly the will to actively resolve and heal old traumas.

## Feelings of guilt

A fundamental distinction must be made between culpability and feelings of guilt.

Anyone who harms, injures or, in extreme cases, murders others is personally culpable. This has consequences: if you turn yourself in or are caught, you will be tried and punished.

If the perpetrator, e.g. a war criminal, does not turn himself in, is not caught or the offence is concealed, then the energy of guilt spreads from the energy field of the perpetrator via the energy field of his family to the coming generations and manifests itself there as an undefined but nonetheless strong feeling of guilt.

Descendants who have not brought any personal culpability upon themselves then have the feeling that they are somehow guilty. In families where the guilt of an ancestor is concealed, there is a tendency to always look for a scapegoat. Someone must be to blame. The blame is shifted back and forth. The accused does not know why he or she should bear any blame. As a result, family members often become divided. At some point, they no longer want to have anything to do with each other.

Of course, the perpetrator may also have feelings of guilt, which in his or her case would be justified. But you are not punished for having guilty feelings without being culpable: the social consensus is that you don't go to prison for that.

However, feelings of guilt, even if they are in no way justified and only inherited from an ancestor, can severely disrupt life. An individual can have the feeling he or she is to blame for everything, even for being ill or for other personal suffering. People who believe themselves to be blameworthy no longer look for the actual causes. Feelings of guilt therefore often make it impossible to find a solution to a stressful situation.

In addition to the fact that we often blame ourselves, we tend to blame others. Frequently, these are the people in our immediate vicinity. This puts partnerships under a strain. Nobody wants to be wrongly blamed, especially not by a loved one. Intimacy is lost.

Feeling guilty drags down your overall life energy. You feel that you are not entitled to a full, rich and happy life. The body cells also sense this. They also cower under the feeling of guilt and do not function as they should. This brings forth symptoms and renders the individual vulnerable to illness.

## Emotional blockages

The energy field completely surrounds and radiates through us with all of its stored and active energies. Every cell in our body and every part of our soul only exists in interaction with the energy field. The blocked emotional energies have an effect at all physical and emotional levels. Each blocked feeling has a particular focus in varying intensity. The organs can be directly affected. This results in different symptoms and illnesses at a mental and physical level.

It therefore makes sense to take a closer look at the various emotional qualities and their specific effects. It is important to realise that every blocked feeling can be passed down through the generations to the youngest born. It does not diminish with the passage of time, but shows its effect with unchecked intensity through the generations. The effects of blocked feelings remain far-reaching in the third and fourth generation and can still be fatal in the youngest generation.

## Blocked love

Blocked love inhibits all expressions of life. The heart in particular reacts to the blockage of love and reflects it on a physical level. Where love cannot flow, there are also blockages to blood flow in the heart. The coronary arteries become constricted. Heart attacks and death can be the result. Or the heart valves calcify and become constricted, which can also lead to severe weakening of the body with fatal consequences. Or a blood clot forms in the heart as an expression of the stagnant energy. If the blood clot then dislodges, it can cause a stroke.

Unresolved conflicts in matters of love can lead to inflammation of the heart muscle, which can significantly restrict the heart's pumping function.

On a psychological level, blocked love leads to a blockage of emotional perception on all levels. Other feelings are also perceived more dully, and the colours take on a grey tinge. The world becomes more unpleasant and remote. The individual becomes isolated, which can lead to total numbness and depression.

The cause of the love blockage is often an unresolved trauma from the past that has been accompanied by unbearable grief.

### Case studies:

The case studies in this book describe the development of symptoms, illnesses and problems as a result of stressful trauma energies in a person's energy field. Knowledge and an understanding of these development mechanisms are the prerequisite for being able to heal with energy medicine.

The case studies in this book do not describe the healing process after a symptom constellation or shamanic healing. Of course, as a doctor, system constellator and shamanic healer, I know from experience that the vast majority of clients benefit significantly from my work, and many even experience complete healing.

But so far, there has not been a statistical survey as part of a study conducted professionally over months and years in the field of symptom constellations in combination with Healing Voices. I therefore see no point in publishing 'success stories' which I am, of course, aware of but which do not really allow the reader to get a clear picture of the enormous healing power of this work. For that, you would also need to know how often it has not helped.

This book can contribute to future scientific studies that quantify the success of the combination of symptom constellations and Healing Voices in verifiable figures.

Nevertheless, the case studies in this book are of great value in their abundance because they open our eyes to the major role that the human energy field plays in the development of illnesses, symptoms and general life problems.

The key details of the case studies have been modified in such a way that they cannot be assigned to a specific case. Most of the examples have several or even many individual cases in their background and represent a distilled essence from a pool of experience.

Nevertheless, the examples describe typical cases as they occur every day in my practice or in my online therapies with clients from all over the world. They are therefore quite normal, everyday cases.

### Family of origin: Love – Great-grandmother

The great-grandparents lose five children as babies. The grief is too much for the great-grandmother. Her heart closes up in these traumas of loss. She no longer feels anything – neither grief nor love. The closed heart is passed on in the family's energy field to the great-granddaughter. She is also unable to feel any grief when she loses two children through miscarriages. Her marriage breaks up. Things don't really work out with new partners either.

### Present family: Angina pectoris – Separation

A couple break up. The man wants to forget because the grief over the loss is too strong. He blocks love through a decision made of his own free will. But a part of his soul has been left behind by the trauma of separation. He knows nothing about it. It is only through heart attacks, which occur years later, that he realises that something is wrong. The blocked love has led to a spasmodic narrowing of his coronary arteries.

### Former life: The petrified heart – The flood

In a past life, a man loses his beloved wife and several children in a catastrophic flood. The grief is overwhelming. His soul freezes in this separation trauma, his heart turns to stone. He no longer feels anything, not even love. Life is over for him. He spends the rest of his days like one of the living dead.

In a later life, the energy of the petrified heart is still in his energy field and mixes with the energy of his new heart. The result is that he has to flee from loving relationships, plus he cannot put any heartfelt energy into his professional career.

## Blocked joy

Blocked joy can lead to a general lack of energy. Many people feel a tightness in their stomach or a reduction in the expression of life that can feel like mild depression. Something is not right – there is a strange feeling of being depressed. Only when these people realise that they have a good reason to be happy can their joy bubble over. Then everything starts to move.

## Blocked grief

Blocked grief means a far-reaching restriction of life energy. Even if the person concerned is not aware of it, grief that cannot flow depresses all cell functions and can therefore lead to a variety of symptoms and illnesses.

The cause of the blockage lies in the mechanisms that kick in during an overwhelming trauma. When the trauma of loss becomes overpowering, a physiological protective mechanism intervenes that ensures pure survival in extreme situations by protecting the body's vital functions from total collapse. All channels of perception are closed down, we no longer notice anything, no longer perceive any feelings. This is not something we do of our own free will or because we have a free choice. It is a primordial, completely unconscious reaction that is automatically triggered when the nervous system is acutely overloaded.

Examples of when grief can lead to trauma freeze include the death of one's own children, partner or other loved ones, especially in the case of sudden deaths due to illness, accidents, natural disasters, war or murder.

For some people, this state of inner numbness persists even after the trauma, especially if no support is forthcoming from those around them. Escape from the reality of the loss leads to a blockage of grief through denial. This leads to inner numbness or even petrification. The individual cannot escape grief wherever he or she goes. It remains in their luggage.

One way of avoiding grief is to rush headlong into imprudent actions. The individual becomes aggressive and looks for someone to blame, someone they can direct their aggression at. Because aggression covers up the grief. Grief disappears behind the anger, which leads to the apportionment of blame. The blame is often unjustified, but it successfully distracts from the grief. The doctor is supposed to be to blame or some other person or even fate or God himself. Some bereaved families fight for years in court in search of someone to blame. For these families, this battle is initially an easier way out than mourning.

Grief is also made impossible when society characterises the death of a loved one as a necessary sacrifice for a 'greater good'. This is the case, for example, when soldiers die in war and the national leadership or the government portray this war as a righteous war of defence. The fallen soldier is then elevated as a hero, placed on a pedestal and taken away from those closest to him. The deeper meaning of mourning, however, is precisely to re-establish the connection to the dead on a spiritual level.

A similar mechanism can be observed in families who have lost someone as a result of a vaccination against coronavirus. These families are also often unable to grieve because the true cause of death has been concealed or presented as a necessary sacrifice to the common good, which is supposedly being safeguarded by the vaccine, despite the death of a daughter or son telling them the opposite.

The blockage of grief has a great disadvantage, even if it offers momentary relief. Because when grief is blocked, love is also blocked and with it the liberating realisation that we can continue to be connected with the lost person on a spiritual level, that love can remain and flow. The blockage of love places a heavy burden on life. The individual becomes depressed. The heart closes up. In extreme cases, it 'turns to stone'. In a less severe form, the individual goes through life feeling depressed, unable to perform to the full extent of their natural ability, and withdraws. In the most severe cases, the individual becomes tired of life and even suicidal.

The suppression of grief also significantly weakens the body's defences. The suppressed grief weighs heavily on the body cells and prevents normal cell function. The result is recurring infections and ultimately serious illnesses such as cancer.

**Case studies:**

### Family of origin: Grief – War crimes

A great-grandfather took part in mass shootings as a soldier in the German Wehrmacht in Russia. The grief for the victims lies in the energy field of the man's family like a lead weight that is unconsciously passed down through the generations and leads to severe depression in the great-granddaughter. She has had suicidal thoughts since childhood. Neither the pills nor the in-patient psychiatric treatment have helped so far.

### Present family: Grief – Lost children

A young couple lose their first two children through miscarriage. They cannot find a common space to grieve for their children. The love for these children is blocked within their hearts. When the next child is born healthy, they no longer think about the lost children. But the blockage in their hearts also has an impact on their relationship as a couple. The intimacy and closeness are lost. They consider separation.

### Past life: Depression – Persecution of witches

In a past life, a woman loses the man she loves. He was persecuted, tortured and murdered as a witch by the henchmen of the Catholic Church. This loss is too much for the woman. Her heart closes. Frozen in grief, she withdraws and no longer takes part in life.

In her current life, she has been depressed since childhood. She has been divorced for years and lives alone. She works well in her professional capacity, but everything is so difficult for her. A part of her soul that should have come over into this life is still stuck in the unresolved trauma of her previous life. This energy is missing in her life.

### Blocked aggression

Wherever healthy anger and aggression cannot flow or manifest itself, there is a congestion of aggression in the energy field of the people involved. The effects of unconsciously blocked aggression can manifest themselves in two fundamentally different ways.

1. **Permanent inhibition** (aggression is invisible)

People who grow up in aggression-inhibited families have no sense of the anger that may be secretly building up inside them. They feel neither anger nor aggression. This means that the development of their own life path is restricted. Because even healthy aggression, which is progressive (aggredere: advance) and takes us forward in the right direction, is blocked. Individuals from such a background have difficulty in defending themselves against attacks of all kinds, are unable to assert their space and position in both their private and professional lives or to find their way in life. They often remain 'victims' of circumstances.

2. **Temporary inhibition** with periodic outbursts of violence (aggression becomes visible)

This can also happen when aggression is blocked. Suddenly, all hell breaks loose. Repeated outbursts of anger in children or violent behaviour and violent crime in adults can be the result.

In families where the level of aggression has been too high for generations, there are frequent outbreaks of verbal or physical violence without any apparent trigger. The true source and the true object of the aggression is often no longer clear after just one generation and so the aggression repeatedly seeks out innocent victims. These may be a partner who is actually loved or even children. Unexplained anger that has been in the family system for generations is a frequent cause of domestic violence.

A man who was sexually abused in a most brutal fashion several times as a child is sitting on a powder keg of aggression, which should actually be directed at the perpetrator, but is instead directed at his wife and child or against himself in the form of drug and alcohol abuse or, in extreme cases, suicide.

On a collective level, armed conflict breaks out against other nations. Repeated hostilities can be traced back to aggression that has festered in the unconscious of society for decades and has its causes in collective traumas of the past such as war, genocide and other mass injustices.

When a society has been repressed for a long time in order to keep unconscious revenge aggression in check, the outbreak of war is sometimes experienced as a liberation. Energy is finally felt again. People feel a surge of strength. Now all they have to do is believe the propaganda that they are fighting for a just cause and soldiers will go joyously to their deaths. This phenomenon was widely observed and documented at the start of the First World War.

Inhibition and the open outbreak of aggression also alternate at a collective level over the course of time.

**Physical consequences of blocked aggression**

Aggression is energy. Energy looks for a way to express itself. When aggression is outwardly blocked, it is instead directed inwards.

On a physical level, auto-aggressive diseases are the result. The body damages itself by directing the immune system against its own tissue and destroying it. This results in allergies, arthritis or 'mysterious' nerve damage such as multiple sclerosis, stomach ulcers (in which stomach acid burns a hole in the stomach wall), cancer (in which the body's own cells degenerate aggressively and destroy the body) and much more besides. Or the individual attracts aggression from outside, such as a car accident.

The indications of hidden aggression in the system are manifold, the symptoms often full of symbolism. For example, polyarthritis of the hands can be an unconscious attempt to keep the murderous potential for aggression in an individual's own energy field in check. To stop himself attempting to grab other people by the throat, he allows his own immune system to destroy his fingers and wrists in recurring bouts of inflammation until his hands freeze in a 'strangulation spasm'.

### Mental consequences of blocked aggression

On a psychological level, blocked aggression leads to depression. This is because, when a strong feeling is blocked, the life energy as a whole is blocked. Depression also acts as a defence against dangerous outbursts of aggression. In order not to kill someone, people prefer to duck and hide under the heavy, powerless cloak of depression

The fact that depression often conceals aggression becomes apparent in suicide, the most obvious auto-aggressive act that a depressed person can commit.

Self-destructive behaviour, self-harm and self-abuse in the form of drug and alcohol addiction are also consequences of blocked aggression.

If the blocked aggression is not directed inwards but breaks through to the outside world, other symptoms become apparent. Even children can show a propensity for violence at school, be repeatedly involved in assaults and fights or react with excessive aggression towards their parents and siblings. In adolescence and adulthood, the risk of antisocial or criminal behaviour increases.

Blocked aggression can be 'inherited' from previous generations of the family or acquired through a personal trauma in childhood or a previous life.

## Blocked aggression in society

On a collective level, blocked aggression also leads to auto-aggressive tendencies. A society whose energy field contains blocked aggression damages or undermines itself in internal battles. In extreme cases, a society dissolves or tears itself apart in a civil war to the point where the state collapses. Entire empires can disintegrate as a result of auto-aggressive mechanisms.

## Murder as a typical example

Two things happen in the victim's energy field during a murder, whether in the private sphere or in the more public context of war crimes. Firstly, defensive aggression builds up in the victim's energy field, which is doomed to be ineffective due to the hopeless situation. Secondly, the unchecked aggression of the perpetrator(s) also passes into the victim's energy field, as the energy fields of the victim and perpetrator come into contact in the course of the crime.

Something similar happens in the offender's energy field, where the blocked defence aggression of the victim and the direct aggression of the perpetrator accumulate.

Because the energy fields of both the victim and the perpetrator are connected to the respective families, this aggression is unconsciously transferred to the energy fields of the families involved and can be passed on to later generations through epigenetic mechanisms.

Because the families from both sides of the crime are part of the state and society, their energy fields are connected to the energy field of society. After collective outbreaks of aggression such as war and genocide, we therefore find blocked aggression in the collective unconscious in all the societies and nations involved, with all its ramifications, which can last for decades or centuries.

**Case studies:**

### Family of origin: Skin rash – The beloved
The great-grandfather fights as a German soldier on the Russian front in the First World War. There he falls in love with a woman who is later murdered in a mass shooting.

In an attempt to forget this trauma of loss, he locks the grief and the revenge aggression against the perpetrators somewhere deep inside. The revenge aggression is passed down through the generations in the family's energy field and leads to an auto-aggressive reaction in the great-grandson in the form of an extremely itchy skin rash that lasts for years.

### Personal trauma: Horror – Sexual abuse
A boy is sexually abused and threatened by several of the nuns in a convent school. As a man, he cannot enter into a sexual relationship with a woman. Before intimate situations can occur, he is overcome by horror. At the same time, the aggression of revenge against the perpetrators radiates from his unconscious to his surroundings and keeps people away from him.

### Former life: Autoimmune disease – Torture
In a previous life, a woman is tortured during Mussolini's fascist dictatorship in Italy in order to force her to betray friends in the resistance. In the end, she is murdered.

The suffering and also the blocked revenge aggression against the perpetrators are stored in her energy field and break through the boundary to the present life. The blocked revenge aggression leads to an auto-aggression disorder in the present life with severe pain in the pelvis and both legs.

## Unrelieved fear

Unrelieved fear in the energy field affects all body cells. They also tremble at a permanently heightened level of fear. Like a person who remains trembling in fear, every cell is also rigid in anticipation of an undefined danger. The functioning of the cell suffers significantly as a result. The muscle cells are weaker, the nerve cells are overstrained and unable to relax, the liver cells work at a slower pace, the intestinal cells absorb less food, the hormone cells produce too little or too much, and the egg and sperm cells are slowed down in their maturation. The physical symptoms triggered by this are varied and can range from chronic fatigue, concentration problems and digestive disorders to infertility and other complaints.

On a psychological level, unrelieved anxiety can cause many symptoms as part of a post-traumatic psychosyndrome. There are many variants ranging from a vague fear of life to a full-blown panic attack with fear of death or the inability to leave the room.

The energetic cause of chronic anxiety is usually an unresolved trauma in the past. After all, anxiety does not come from nowhere, but has a root cause. Treatment therefore begins with a search for the original trauma.

## Case studies:

### Family of origin: Panic attack – Rape
A woman is raped by Russian soldiers at the end of the Second World War. Her mother and her sister intervene and are shot on the spot. The trauma settles in the unconscious energy field of the family. The fear is passed down through the generations. The granddaughter regularly develops panic attacks when she gets involved in an intimate relationship with a man.

**Present family: Fear of love – Fatal heart attack**

A man in his mid-forties suffers a sudden cardiac arrest at work. In the trauma of sudden death, his soul is frozen in a permanent state of agony.

For his wife, his death is a trauma of loss. A part of her soul freezes in the shock of grief, isolates itself and somehow feels cut off from all areas of life. Even after twenty years, she remains alone. She feels abandoned and does not enter into a new partnership. Unconsciously, she is afraid of losing a new partner again through early death. She would rather remain alone. But in the depths of her heart she is dissatisfied.

**Past life: No boundaries – The Inquisition**

In a past life in the Middle Ages, a woman is persecuted, tortured and murdered as a witch by the Catholic Inquisition. The massive violation of boundaries through rape, torture and murder becomes fixed in this woman's energy field in the sense of a trauma freeze. The horror and fear break through the energy boundary to the present incarnation and emerge as an unconscious burden. The client is unable to set healthy boundaries. The fear carried over from the torture in the previous life makes this impossible.

The result is failed relationships and a chronic overload at work, because the client cannot say no and takes on too many jobs.

## Mental attachment formed by foreign souls

In addition to the burdens carried over from trauma suffered by family members or by the individual him/herself, energies from other people can also flow into that person's energy field. These are the souls of people who actually have no connection with the person to whom they become attached. Nor do they belong to the family or to a previous incarnation. They are usually the souls of deceased persons who have attached themselves to certain places: houses, plots of land or even locations in the wild where something traumatic such as a battle or an accident has occurred. If an individual arrives in such a place, spends a night there or even moves in and lives there, these psychic energies can attach themselves to this newcomer and occupy him or her. A person to whom something like this happens suddenly has negative feelings that they never had before, such as inexplicable anger, fear and sadness. Or they develop nightmares or, when awake, feel that there is someone else in the room or lurking behind a curtain. Such individuals are often declared insane, put on antidepressant medication or admitted to a psychiatric institution. But nothing gets better as a result.

I remember a young man who sought my help because he had been suffering from anxiety for months, especially at night in the apartment he had moved into six months earlier. He sometimes felt the presence of a man waiting for him on the basement stairs with a long knife. As soon as he fell asleep, he had nightmares of being stabbed and bleeding to death, watching the murderer wipe the knife on the tablecloth so that it was clean for the next victim.

He had been on sick leave for eight weeks and had been on an odyssey from psychiatrist to psychiatrist. The medication didn't help, nor did the conversations. Behavioural therapy came to nothing. He was diagnosed as mentally ill. Nobody considered the possibility that the young man felt an energy that was actually present, which was acting on him from the outside through a mental possession and did not emanate from a disturbed inner self. Mental

87

possession does not feature in the training of psychiatrists and psychotherapists.

In the symptom constellation, in addition to the fear and the message of fear, I actually brought a representative for the man that the client felt in his apartment. The information from these few positions clearly showed that the client was indeed possessed by a foreign soul. It was directly behind him, in the centre of his energy field.

Effective treatment of mental possession is possible with the help of Healing Voices. In the case described, the shamanic healing energies sent the soul of the stranger away to the souls to which he really belonged, away into a liberating light where he had been awaited in vain for a long time. The young man was then completely free of this burden. He even stayed in the apartment for a few more months without the anxiety or nightmares returning.

Most people who suffer from schizophrenia are affected by mental possession. However, occupation by foreign souls is rather rare. In most cases, the souls that attach themselves in schizophrenia originate from the family system or a traumatic experience in a previous incarnation.

## Disturbance by the collective energy field

An individual's personal energy field is closely connected to the collective energy fields of society, the nation and humanity. The emotional energies that spread collectively in a society can carry all the qualities of personal feelings such as joy, aggression, anger, hate, fear, sadness or revenge. The difference here is that many people are exposed to these feelings at the same time, often without realising where they have come from.

At the height of the coronavirus pandemic, for example, many people sat in their own homes and were afraid, not because there was an actual threat, but because millions of people in society were afraid, all at the same time. The collective fear became tangible as personal fear.

Depressive feelings can also spread collectively in a similar way. A depressed society also affects the personal well-being of individual citizens without there being a personal cause.

Anger and hatred that has built up in society can suddenly erupt simultaneously in many people who previously felt neither anger nor hatred.

At the beginning of the First World War, a strange enthusiasm for war gripped millions of people in just a few days. Among them were many men who had previously been avowed pacifists. They too were overwhelmed by the collective feeling of enthusiasm for the war. One prominent example is Carl Zuckmayer, who experienced this phenomenon himself and described it in his autobiography *A Part of Myself.*

It is important to understand that collective feelings are primarily indistinguishable from personal feelings. We ask ourselves, what is wrong with me today, and we look for the cause in our personal life. Sometimes, however, the answer lies on a collective level. Behind it are social events such as collective trauma, especially war, oppression, collective manipulation, marginalisation of minorities, social injustice and so on.

The first step in freeing ourselves from stressful, collective energies and feelings is to recognise that the feelings we are experiencing are collective. This is already enough to bring some relief; it's not me personally who is aggressive, but the increased level of aggression is collective, it is in society. I am not personally sad; I just feel the sadness that lies like a blanket over society. The hatred that I feel is not my own personal hatred; it is the hatred of society. It has nothing to do with me personally.

If we realise that, we no longer need to expend energy and worry to find out why we feel this way. It's a collective process.

Even if this realisation allows us to keep the stressful, collective feelings at arm's length to some extent, many other people who are unaware of these connections are still fully exposed to them. We therefore continue to live in an anxiety-ridden society in which fear can turn into aggression at any time.

In order to achieve a fundamental improvement on a collective level, people would ideally have to get together to find out where the collective causes of the problem lie. Collective system constellations are an excellent tool for this. By recognising the collective causes of a social burden, an improvement in the situation can already be achieved. Political and social consequences can already be drawn at this point.

If the cause is a collective trauma from the past, as is often the case, a healing impulse on the collective soul level is needed in addition to the revelatory work in the collective constellation. This is achieved in a striking and powerful way with the shamanic healing energies of Healing Voices. You can find video recordings of collective healings of socially relevant problem areas on my homepage at: www.dr-rauscher.de/en/kollektive-aufstellung

# Chapter 3: Diagnosis

A guiding principle that medical students learn at university is: "God has placed the diagnosis before the therapy." In other words, the doctor or therapist must first find out where the patient's symptoms are coming from and what illness lies behind them. The doctors must therefore make a diagnosis and give the illness a name so that they know exactly what they are treating. The more precisely the doctor knows how the illness has arisen, the greater the chance that he or she will choose the right treatment method.

When making a diagnosis, Western conventional medicine is content to find the illness on a purely material, physical level. This is where efforts to diagnose with maximum accuracy already come to a halt. The energetic causes of illnesses, which are located in the human energy field and from there have a constant effect on the body, are not investigated for the simple reason that doctors and scientists trained at Western universities generally know nothing about them.

This gap can be closed by energy medicine, which deals precisely with this phenomenon. For the energy medicine practitioner, the diagnosis is only complete when the energetic cause of the physical or mental illness has also been found. Because there is always an energetic cause. Knowing it opens up completely new treatment options that usefully complement conventional medical therapies.

The best diagnostic tool in energy medicine is the system constellation. It is the energy medicine practitioner's equivalent of the MRI machine. It can be used to 'X-ray' the energy field as well as the physical structures. Unlike with an MRI, practitioner and patient also receive detailed information about the function of the constellated organ. In a conventional medical setting, this would require additional, sometimes complicated examinations and tests.

## The system constellation as a diagnostic tool

System constellations were developed around forty years ago by Bert Hellinger, a German family therapist, in the form of family constellations, and became accessible to a wider professional and lay audience following the publication of his book *Love's Hidden Symmetry* (German title: *Zweierlei Glück*) in 1993. Therapists all over the world now work with family constellations. There are countless books by Bert Hellinger and other authors that have been translated into many languages.

It was soon discovered that the constellation method could be successfully applied not only to family systems, but also to other systems. When a family is constellated, this is called a family constellation. When the organ system of the body is constellated, it is called organ constellation. If you constellate symptoms or problems, this is called symptom constellation or problem constellation. When you constellate professional systems (i.e. an organisation or a company), this is called organisational constellation or systemic business coaching. 'System constellation' is the umbrella term for all these forms of constellation.

The methodological core of every system constellation is always the same. It makes it possible to obtain valuable and otherwise barely accessible information about the interrelationships of the system concerned. In order to understand how information acquisition works in a system constellation, you need to know the following:

The information about each person's state of mind, including their relationships with other people, both living and deceased, lies in the air in an invisible form, as if in a special Wi-Fi field. Information about traumatic events that happened decades or centuries ago can also be found in this information field.

In addition, information about connections in organisations and companies and global collective systems such as ecosystems and economic and financial systems are stored there.

The system constellation gives us access to this huge, comprehensive pool of information. It gives us an immense advantage today compared to past times when this access was not possible.

Thanks to the use of technical Wi-Fi fields, we are now accustomed to the idea that masses of information can surround us in invisible form. The concept is no longer anything special. Even though we cannot perceive with our five senses how millions of websites, millions of mobile phone calls and thousands of television and radio programmes are 'hidden away' between the air molecules, we still happily use the Wi-Fi fields every day. All we need is a technical receiver, a smartphone, a laptop or a television set.

It is to Bert Hellinger's credit that he made two especially important discoveries: firstly, the discovery that the information field described above exists; and secondly, that there is also a receiver for this information field and that we humans can be this receiver. With our intuitive ability to perceive, we have the possibility of gaining access to all of this information.

However, it does not happen when we simply sit around drinking coffee. A certain framework is needed for the information to flow. This framework is called a system constellation.

As with the technical reception of Wi-Fi information from the internet, certain requirements must also be met for the system constellation so that the information can flow.

If you want to receive Wi-Fi with a laptop, you must first ensure that power is available via battery or mains. Then all parts of the laptop must work together correctly and nothing must be broken. Then you type in the internet address, dial the telephone number or tune in to the radio station. You have to tell the device from which area within the huge information pool of the internet it is supposed to receive information. Only then will you hear the right radio station, see the right website displayed or be connected to the right telephone number.

**The framework**

This is no different with system constellations, which provide the framework for receiving information from the human energy field. The following conditions are necessary and must be met:

1. The system positions must be set up in relation to each other. The framework must be stretched so that the relationships between the positions can be shown.

2. A person must mentally determine who or what a position stands for. This adjusts the reception channel. The corresponding action would be selecting a radio station or typing a website address into a web browser. In a family constellation, for example, it must be clear whether a position stands for the father, the mother or the child. A single person must define this. That is enough. Numerous research constellations have shown that no other group member, not even the constellation facilitator, needs to know which position stands for whom. In most constellations, everybody knows for whom or what the positions stand, but it is not necessary in ensuring that the channel is opened and information flows.

3. The representatives who stand on a position must do so voluntarily. If someone feels pressurised to do so, this person is not free and open to perform the function of a 'radio receiver'.

4.  The representatives in the positions should be impartial. All ideas about how they might feel in this position should be dropped. Such preconceptions play no role and would only disturb. In practice, this proviso is not a problem, as the information from the 'Knowing Field' feels somewhat different to the ideas the representatives have in their mind. Most representatives can easily distinguish this after the second or third experience.

If the systemic constellation takes place in a therapy or coaching group, the positions are filled by group members. As soon as the representatives stand in the positions, the information begins to flow. Specifically, the representatives feel the way the person they represent is feeling mentally or physically.

When a person who has already died is assigned a position in a constellation, the representative feels the way the soul of the deceased person feels at that moment.

At this point, it is important to realise that we can never look into the past with a constellation, but can only ever grasp the present moment. This also applies to the state of mind of the souls of deceased persons. From this we can conclude that the souls continue to exist after the body has been shed and take all feelings and even internalised attitudes with them. The emotions do not go to the grave with the corpse, but remain with the soul, wherever the souls may go after death. To better understand these connections, you can detach the term 'soul' from all religious concepts. It is essentially simple. You are a soul, I am a soul, everyone is a soul. We have the body for a while, then we shed it. After that, we are still the same soul, we have feelings somehow and have multiple connections.

Basically, that is the good news. Because if you know that, with a constellation, we always look into the present moment (i.e. into the present state of the souls of the living and the dead), then you can also understand that mental states can change while we are working with them today. Otherwise this would not be understandable. Because what happened yesterday or a hundred years ago cannot be changed. However, the current state of mind of the souls involved can very well change.

When a representative stands in a non-personal system position, such as a symptom, a disease or a department of an organisation, they begin to feel the way this position 'feels'. This is not meant literally here, because non-personal system positions are not people. They do not feel, but they do have a state of being that carries information. Since the representative is a human being and can only receive information at the feeling level, the information about the non-personal position is apparently transferred automatically (through an unknown transmitter process) to the human feeling level. It is then relatively straightforward to intuitively deduce from these sensations the 'state of mind' or rather the state of the non-personal positions and to understand what they mean in a figurative sense. Of course, it is helpful if you have a basic knowledge of the non-personal position. For example, if you want to categorise information coming from the organ position 'heart', it is an advantage if you know the anatomy and functioning of the heart. If you want to interpret the information coming from the system position 'Company X', it is an advantage if you know the basic structure and the products or services of this company.

In individual therapy or individual coaching, I have slips of paper placed on the floor on which the name of the person or the name of the non-personal system position is written. The slips of paper are only placeholders so that it is clear to everyone where the positions are located. The actual work, in which information also flows in the individual setting, begins when I stand in the positions one after the other as a representative and collect the information from these positions.

# The flow of information

The representatives in a system constellation receive the information from the knowing field in five ways:

1. Physical sensations (pain, cold, heat)
2. Mental sensations (feelings, moods)
3. Movement impulses (gestures, change of position)
4. Words, sentences and insights that are 'in the air'
5. Sounds, images or cinematic scenes in the mind's eye

### Examples of physical sensations:
Pressure on the heart, pain in the spine, headaches, dizziness, physical weakness, joint pain, well-being, feeling of weight on the shoulders, a clenched fist and much more besides.

### Examples of emotional sensations:
Joy, sadness, depression, fear, shame, loneliness, isolation, aggression, loving feelings, connectedness, feelings of repulsion or attraction and much more besides.

### Examples of movement impulses and gestures:
Moving to another place, sitting down, lying down, standing up, kneeling down, standing up tall, pressing lips together (secret), making a fist (aggression), crossing arms, opening arms, protective posture with both hands in a certain direction, hugging, retreating, wandering gaze as if looking for something, hands searching for something on or in the ground or an outstretched arm with a finger pointing (accusation).

### Examples of sentences and insights that are 'in the air':
Words, sentences and insights are sometimes on the lips of the representatives, but also come to the attention of the facilitator.

Suddenly there is a sentence and you intuitively know that this sentence is important in the constellation. Here is a small selection from many:

"In such a situation, you must be going mad", "Someone's missing", "There's a secret here" etc.

### Examples of images or scenes 'in the mind's eye':

- You see yourself in a prison or as a long-term inmate in a psychiatric ward
- You see mass graves with many dead in front of you
- You can see a battlefield with trenches (First World War)
- You stand with many others with your back to a wall just before a mass shooting
- You see bombs falling, debris everywhere. Or you sit in an aeroplane and look down, where the people are very small.
- and much more besides.

### Examples of sounds and noises:

Sounds and noises can be heard by the 'mind's ear', but often also come from the immediate or more distant surroundings of where the constellation is taking place, i.e. they are real noises that obviously fit in with what is happening in the constellation. For example:

- The sound of a rock band on the neighbouring lawn becomes the thunder of bombs hitting the ground in World War II.
- The high-pitched sound of an organ pipe being tuned and lasting for minutes becomes a siren announcing a bombing raid
- Church bells accompany the reconciliation of a couple.

- The siren of a passing ambulance indicates that the constellation could be about an accident
- and much more besides.

### The Symptom Constellation

Every form of systemic constellation serves the diagnostic function. An attempt is made to find out where the original trauma lies that has led to the problem presented.

In conventional family constellations, the cause is sought in the family of origin or present family. Other areas such as personal trauma in childhood or a previous incarnation are often not taken into consideration.

To take all four of these areas into account, I have developed a special form of constellation work that I call **Symptom Constellation.**

I focus on the symptom, the illness or the problem. In the next step, I address the central question of which of the four major areas is causing the burden. To do this, I carry out the 'four-column test'. Because the first step is always the diagnosis. The symptom constellation is characterised by the fact that, unlike a classic family constellation, it also opens up all other important areas as possible causes.

### The four-column test

I perform the four-column test at an early stage of the symptom constellation. Before I start the test, I first set up three positions:

- the client
- the symptom, the disease or the problem presented
- the message of the symptom, disease or problem

The 'Message' position is very important because it often provides much more information from the energetic background than the symptom or the disease itself.

After these positions have revealed their information from the Knowing Field, I begin the test.

To repeat: there are basically four sources of stressful, disease-inducing energies:

1. A trauma in the family of origin that a member of a previous generation has suffered or inflicted on other people. Parents, grandparents or great-grandparents are often involved. This is the most common case. About 60% of my clients show this energetic background.

2. A trauma in the present family. This is the family of which you are the founder. Members are past, present or future love partners and your own children, including deceased, miscarried or aborted children.

3. A trauma that you yourself have experienced in this life, in childhood, adolescence or adulthood.

4. A trauma that you have experienced yourself, but not in this life, rather in a previous life. Every person has many previous incarnations. The unresolved traumas of previous incarnations are energetically inscribed in a person's energy field. Depending on the current life situation, these traumas can also cause symptoms, illnesses or other problems. This is quite common. More than 30% of my clients show this energetic background to their problems.

To represent **the first column**, I define a position somewhere in the outer area of the constellation, call it 'Family of Origin' and step into this position as a representative. It does not stand for one person, but a pool that includes all family members: parents, siblings, grandparents and all ancestors. Now it becomes clear whether this area has a connection to the current problem. As a rule, one of the following four reactions will occur:

- the right arm points to the problem and thus indicates a connection to the father's side

- the left arm points to the problem and thus indicates a connection to the mother's side
- both arms are raised and point towards the problem. In this case, the energetic load is on both sides.
- a gesture that means "No, I'm not connected". This is often a shrug of the shoulders or a shake of the head. In this case, the cause of the problem does not lie in the family of origin.

Now you already know whether the family of origin is involved. You also know whether it is the father's side, the mother's side or both.

But even if the family of origin shows a connection to the current problem, I continue with the test because sometimes there are double stresses from different areas. This is rare, but it does happen. A typical case of double stress occurs, for example, when a previous incarnation was shared with a parent of the current life and both the client and the parent were involved in the original trauma of the previous incarnation.

**The second column** tests 'Present Family'. I choose a different place in the outer circle of the constellation for each column.

The reactions that show up in this position vary, but show either a connection or no connection to the problem.

**The third column** is a personal trauma in this life, in childhood, adolescence or later. I define this position as 'Client's Personal Trauma in this Lifetime' that may have a connection to the current problem. It is important to name this position precisely.

This basically applies to every item in a constellation. The positions should be named as precisely as possible so that you do not receive confusing, overly broad information from the information field.

The reactions that show up in the position of a personal trauma also vary and indicate either a connection or no connection to the problem.

In **the fourth column,** I test 'Client's Past Life' that may have a connection to the current problem.

This part of the test is important because unresolved traumas in previous incarnations are the second most common cause of problems after Family of Origin.

The reactions shown in this position also vary and show either a connection or no connection to the problem. An arm is often raised here too to indicate a connection. As it is often an aggressive trauma that has ended the previous life, aggression may already be evident in this position.

If none of these columns respond, I test 'Professional Situation' as **the fifth column.** An unresolved problem at work can also trigger symptoms of all kinds. This is comparatively rare in a therapeutic situation. In business coaching, however, this is a frequent occurrence.

There are also other rare areas or situations that can lead to symptoms or problems, e.g. mental possession by the soul of a deceased stranger (very rare) or an energetic burden from souls that are bound to a place, a house, a farm or a landscape (somewhat more common). I only test these areas if there are definite indications or if the four-column test has shown a negative result in the four main areas.

If you follow the above procedure, it will be easy for you to integrate and apply the four-column test in the constellations you lead. After the test, in the vast majority of cases you will know to which of these areas the original trauma and therefore the energetic cause of the problem can be assigned.

Now you can ask the client specific questions about the area involved. What happened in the family of origin or present family? Was there a trauma in childhood?

If a previous incarnation is causally involved, questions to the client do not lead anywhere, because the client usually knows nothing about the previous life. The trauma and the people or events involved are only revealed in the constellation. This requires detective work to uncover step by step how the unresolved trauma in the past life is connected to the client's symptom.

Once the diagnosis has been made and the connection between the symptom, illness or problem and the underlying trauma has become clear, the therapy can follow.

# Chapter 4: Therapy in energy medicine

Therapy in energy medicine is aimed at diminishing or completely eliminating the pathogenic influence of the stressful emotional energies that emanate from the energy field and which affect a person's organs and soul.

Once the triggering trauma has been identified in the diagnostic stage with the aid of a symptom constellation, the next steps are about creating the right conditions for healing to occur. An important part of healing is the transformation of an unresolved trauma into a resolved state, so that the trauma and all its stressful consequences can finally be consigned to the past. This can be achieved with the methods of energy medicine.

## Basic healing methods of energy medicine

A wide variety of methods are used in energy medicine around the world. In my work extending over many decades, two treatment methods have proven to be effective. They support and complement each other. One is symptom constellation and the other is shamanic healing energies.

## Symptom constellations

In addition to their diagnostic function, symptom constellations also have a therapeutic effect. As a method for obtaining information, they provide important insights into the energetic background of the disorder. The clients learn exactly where the energetic cause of their symptoms lies. Knowledge of how everything is connected comes as a relief in itself and has a healing effect. The truth heals.

If you learn, for example, that the depressive burden actually belongs to your grandmother who died in the war, the burden can already recede from your own person and move in the direction of your grandmother. The mood lightens within minutes.

Or if it becomes clear that a skin rash with itching goes back to a previous incarnation in which the client was burnt at the stake, this realisation can cause the symptom to be released and move energetically in the direction of the previous incarnation.

These are incipient healing developments that begin as early as the initial phase of the constellation. However, in order for the healing development to completely reach its destination, further information needs to flow. For example, the circumstances of a trauma must be clarified, thereby expanding the client's awareness, which is crucial at this point. Clients must know about the connections in which they find themselves. In the symptom constellation, this is made possible by bringing in the people involved in the trauma step by step. This shines more and more light on what is happening until a sufficiently clear picture of the events emerges.

The burdensome energy is already beginning to leave the client. An energetic decoupling of the burdensome energy from the client's energy field takes place. The activating factor for this healing development at this point is indeed the expansion of consciousness.

## Consciousness

The term is used in two ways.

On the one hand, we speak of consciousness, which can be lost in the event of traumatic brain injury, cardiac arrest or anaesthesia. You are unconscious and no longer have any sensory perception until you regain consciousness. This is not the type of consciousness at issue here.

In our context, it is the second meaning of this term which applies, namely the consciousness that is formed when we come to a realisation, i.e. we know something for certain and are also able to comprehend how that which we observe is connected and related. The expansion of this type of consciousness plays a central role in healing processes. In order to be healed, we have to recognise something beyond doubt and also understand the connections between what we have recognised and life as a whole.

In the following, I use the term 'consciousness' exclusively in the sense of this latter definition.

Life offers us the opportunity to expand our consciousness step by step. Perhaps this is even the real meaning of life. Creation becomes aware of itself through the medium of human consciousness. We are part of the universe, just as a grain of sand is part of the beach, or a drop of water is part of the sea. In order to completely fulfil our part in the 'concert' of the greater whole, the expansion of consciousness is ingrained into our being as a necessity from the very beginning. It is our role to recognise who we are in the interplay of all parts of this world. In doing so, every step towards realising our own being will repeatedly go beyond the limits of our current consciousness. What we have known so far is replaced by a new knowledge that provides a larger framework for recognising ourselves and the world. The broader our consciousness becomes through the accumulation of knowledge, the more complete and healthier we become. One of the most important elements of a growing consciousness is the realisation that we are deeply connected to everything external and everything internal, indeed that we as human beings are defined by our connections and only exist through them.

Because we humans like to operate within our comfort zone, we need external events to expand our consciousness. Life provides us with such events, but they are often unpleasant. Problems, symptoms or illnesses appear out of nowhere and scare us out of our comfort zone, alerting us to the need to expand our consciousness. We are obliged to recognise the nature of our inner selves and allow it to grow in order to remain or become healthy.

Despite intensive research, it has not yet been possible to clarify what consciousness actually is. We do not know where it is located, what form it takes, nor how it is connected to us. The assumption that consciousness is located in the brain is pure conjecture, for which there is no evidence whatsoever.

When we realise and accept that we humans are beings made up of pure energy – and this book is my contribution to bringing this knowledge into the world – then it becomes more and more probable that consciousness is not located in the physical structures of the brain, but outside the body in the energy fields that surround and permeate us. Because these energy fields are connected with all other energy fields, basically with the entire universe, it is difficult to imagine at this point that there could be such a thing as a personal consciousness at all. Because when we as individuals expand our consciousness and this expansion happens in our personal energy field, then other people, other energy beings, perhaps even whole collectives become aware of something. Conversely, it is possible that we experience impulses and energy inflows from the energy fields of other people or from the great energy field of the universe, which change and expand our consciousness.

The actual significance of a symptom is the expansion of consciousness, which enables us to reconnect with people close to us who have been separated by fate, or to reconnect with parts of our own soul that have been left behind in past traumas. This expansion of consciousness is made possible by the information that flows through the symptom constellation. In this way, the actual meaning of the symptom is taken into account. The decoupling of the burdensome energies from the client's energy field, as described above, is already the first healing effect of this expansion of consciousness.

## Healing sentences

In order to bring expanded consciousness into the relationships, words, phrases and sentences are used in the symptom constellation that can be said to a partner, parents, grandparents or similar. These are the famous 'healing sentences' that Bert Hellinger regularly made use of in family constellations. These are sentences that are usually 'hanging in the air' in the final phase of a family constellation, are recognised by the constellation facilitator and suggested to the client as a possibility. It is often about clarifying the relationship or the ritual return of an energetic burden to a previous generation. The spoken word, if it can be spoken honestly and with inner conviction, has a connecting and healing effect on the relationship.

### Typical healing sentences are:

**Child to parents:** "Dear mum, dear dad, I have tried to carry your burden out of love. But it's too heavy for my small shoulders. Because I am only your daughter/son. Yes, I'm happy to be that. But from now on, I will respectfully and lovingly leave your burden entirely with you."

**In a couple relationship:** "I brought something difficult from my family into our relationship. I didn't know about it myself. I have done you wrong. None of this has anything to do with you. I'm sorry that I blamed you for it. I'm trying to make that up to you."

These are just examples. Healing sentences are multifaceted, do not follow a template and are adapted to the situation in the constellation. They are frequently used in classic family constellations. They often succeed and have a healing effect. Sometimes they do not succeed and have no effect. This is because the original trauma has not really been resolved at this stage of the constellation, because the souls of the people who experienced it are still stuck in the trauma freeze. In this case, the use of a healing sentence to hand back an adopted burden is either not successful or only partially so.

In a symptom constellation, I therefore always try to resolve the original trauma. This is possible with the second method of energy medicine, namely shamanic-energetic healing. After this, healing sentences are usually no longer necessary, because the souls of those affected have been freed from the original trauma and there is no longer any burden for the client to carry on as a descendant. Alternatively, the healing sentences can now be spoken with inner conviction, only now manifesting their healing effect.

## Shamanic-energetic healing energies

The shamans of this world work with invisible healing energies. These healing energies are present everywhere and at all times in an invisible form in the air, like in a special Wi-Fi field. The methods of the various shamanic traditions differ in form. Some shamans use objects and animal totems, while others heal with gestures, drums and chants. However, the healing energy that flows through these actions always has the same source: the 'healing energy field' that surrounds us at all times, no matter where we are.

As you can read in much of the relevant literature, the shaman normally chooses his students and summons them. From a traditional point of view, it is not enough if the potential trainee feels the desire to train as a shaman. He or she must be called or summoned. If the chosen ones do not answer this call, they generally fall ill, sometimes deathly ill. In order to become well again, there is no choice but to follow the call, serve as an apprentice with a shaman for years and go through a rigorous and time-consuming training programme.

The training is necessary because the students must be prepared for the task of making themselves available as mediums for shamanic healing energies. The shaman is a mediator between the worlds, between the healing energies and the human being. As a medium, the shaman makes his body and his voice available to the healing energies. Whatever additional tools he uses, invisible healing energies flow through all his actions, gestures and chants. It is essential that the medium is free from human preconceptions or selfish desires so that the healing energies are not distorted or clouded as they flow through the medium.

The shamanic students must learn to reduce their ego as much as possible, ideally to dissolve it completely. To do this, they look into their own shadow world, get to know their own shadows and banish them with the help of the healing teacher. Only then is it guaranteed that their healing activities will not be disturbed by the shadow side of their soul. This is a demanding task and can only be achieved under the guidance of an experienced healer.

In cultures where archaic shamanic traditions have died out, the vocation of shamanic healer can also take a different route. The shamans who were able to pass on the healing tradition from generation to generation no longer exist in many countries. In these cultures, the healing energy field sometimes selects candidates directly without the mediation of a traditional shaman. Such a candidate is prepared for the call from the healing energy field by life, professional experience and sometimes hard personal crises, without knowing it and without wanting it. When a candidate is mature, he or she will suddenly have contact with the healing energy. This can happen in very different ways, but it is always impressive and surprising. The call comes out of nowhere.

That's exactly what happened to me in 2001.

### The call to become a shaman

At that time, I was already a specialist in internal medicine, a systemic therapist and a trainer in systemic constellations. Together with my wife, I ran a seminar house in Bavaria, surrounded by meadows, forests and mountains. A number of shamans used our seminar house to perform shamanic healing rituals with their groups. Of course, as the tenant of the property, I participated in all those workshops. As a doctor and psychotherapist, I was interested in how shamans heal. I experienced healing rituals in the Native American medicine wheel and sweat lodges.

Three years later, I was already an initiated sweat lodge leader. But the thought of healing with shamanic energies myself was far from my mind.

Until a certain day in midsummer…

The stones were already glowing hot in the embers of the fire. I sat on a tree stump and watched the fire master leaning on a gardening fork and looking into the glowing coals. It would soon be time for the sweat lodge to begin.

I lit sage in a clam shell, let the flames flare up briefly and then blew them out. White smoke rose up in fine wisps. At the entrance to the sweat lodge, the participants waited in a long line, each clad only in a large towel, so that I could purify them one by one with sage smoke. This is what the Native American sweat lodge ceremony is all about: physical, emotional and spiritual cleansing so that blocked energy can flow. It can be painful at the places where the blockages are located. Sooner or later, the humid heat pushes people to their limits. A sweat lodge can last several hours.

As the leader of the sweat lodge, I sat just to the right of the entrance. The hut arched over us like an igloo, like a womb with only one exit. Almost thirty people were sitting on the grass floor, still cool at that point, around the pit in the centre. Now the fire master brought glowing stones into the hut and dropped them into the hollow in the centre. After the seventh stone I signalled to him that it was enough. He released and dropped the blankets suspended above the entrance. Immediately we were surrounded by darkness. The stones glowed in the centre.

I poured on three ladles of water. The water evaporated with a loud hiss. The hut filled with hot steam. I began to beat the drum quietly. The first round had begun. It serves to set the mood. The participants have undergone long preparation and know that they can use their voice freely in the first round, that they can utter sounds. Most of them are not used to letting their voice be heard. The first blockages are at throat level. But with the beat of the drum, the didgeridoo blown by a friend and a few brave people following my high notes, a polyphonic song without words soon unfolded quietly and carefully.

Whenever energy starts to flow, even if it is only the voice that dares to emit it, other blockages are also stimulated, tension in the neck, blocked grief in the stomach, blocked love in the heart as well as anger and pain. Energy that is stimulated throbs against the walls behind which it is imprisoned. It wants to flow, wants to connect, wants to show itself and exert an effect.

That is why we make sounds in the first round of the sweat lodge, that is why we sit in the heat, with only the darkness in front of us, on which our own souls are reflected.

I had often been present and experienced this before a shaman initiated me as a sweat lodge leader. In my work as a systemic facilitator, I had already learnt beforehand to let go of any preconceptions, to become completely permeable to information from the invisible field, to information that often communicates itself intuitively as a feeling, sometimes with words, whole sentences or even inner images. It's like being in the cinema. The invisible is projected on the blank screen of intuitive perception. But nothing had prepared me for what was to happen that day in the sweat lodge.

I had already attended many shamanic healing ceremonies and sometimes found healing in them myself. But I had never been through a shamanic teaching. No shaman had chosen me as his disciple, told me that a higher power wanted me to become a shaman. No one had prepared me.

On that day in the sweat lodge, we initially had the impression of a distant whale song, but soon our voices swelled and became powerful and loud. Suddenly my singing changed. Consonants and vowels were blended into the initially pure and smooth tones. It sounded like an archaic language. Soon I was no longer singing, but speaking in a language that was foreign to me. The words made no sense to my head, but abundant sense to my innermost soul and heart. I simply gave in to the impulses, as I had learnt to do. My mind was just an observer. But I was amazed to hear how the words turned into complete sentences. I no longer had any doubt that someone was speaking through me to the whole group. The people sitting around in the sweat lodge fell silent. All you could hear was the wind in the trees at the edge of the nearby forest, the crackling of the fire and the strange words that came from my lips in all kinds of tones. Suddenly someone was sobbing at the back of the sweat lodge. Rows of participants began to weep, some quietly, others burst into tears. Long-suffered pain broke through. My voice grew stronger, drowned out even the loudest weeping, continued to speak to the group and only became softer when, one after the other, they calmed down.

Never before had I experienced such an opening of the emotional worlds in the first round. When it was completely quiet in the hut, I pulled back the blanket at the entrance. It was time for the first break, fresh air blew in, the fire master passed bottles of water into the hut. New hot stones were brought in. Then the blanket was dropped again. The next three rounds were quieter, almost more peaceful than usual.

The sweat lodge session ended with us being showered with a garden hose. Afterwards, when we were all sitting around the fire in our clothes again, one of the participants asked me:

"What was that?" Everybody knew what he meant.

"I don't know," I said. "I really don't know."

### Healing Voices

In the days that followed, this experience naturally preoccupied me. I had already realised that I had become a medium for healing energy. As voices and sounds played an important role in this, I also had a name for it: Healing Voices! It had felt good and many participants in the group had obviously benefited from it. But should I really also be doing shamanic work? I was already a doctor, systemic therapist and trainer, so I thought, please don't expect me to become a shaman as well! No, that was too much for me. Apart from my role as a sweat lodge leader, I had never experienced a shamanic initiation. I felt no entitlement and, to be honest, no desire to continue being a medium for shamanic healing energies. It must have been a one-off thing, maybe even a great moment of healing but nothing more. That's what I thought at the time.

For several years, I refused to pursue this phenomenon any further. I would certainly not employ the method in my medical practice. When it came to treating illnesses in my family, however, I had fewer reservations. I successfully treated cardiac arrhythmia, pain and inflammation of artificial hips and knee joints in members of my family. These few experiences, which were spread over several years, convinced me of the effectiveness of Healing Voices. But my refusal to use this method professionally continued.

Until one day in Provence I fell off my bike. In a state of semi-consciousness, I realised immediately that I had sunstroke. It was a hot day. As I was wearing a head covering and was equipped with a plentiful supply of water, the ten kilometres I had ridden on a flat route couldn't really be the cause. But there was no time for such considerations. My wife was only twenty metres away in the tourist information office. She had no idea that I was lying in the car park next to my bike, close to passing out. I grabbed the water bottle and drank a litre and a half as quickly as I could. A fluid intake would surely fix my circulation problem, I thought. But it wasn't that simple. Although I was lying on the ground, my eyes kept going black. I crawled a few metres to a nearby park bench and put my feet up. Above me, white clouds drifted across the deep blue sky of Provence. Who would tell my wife that I had been taken unconscious to a clinic by an ambulance crew? Where had she even been for so long?

My condition slowly improved. When my wife finally arrived after a quarter of an hour, I was already sitting up again, resting my back against the park bench. I hadn't needed emergency treatment after all. After consuming another litre of cool water, I was well enough to cycle the three hundred metres to the new hotel, albeit with very weak legs.

It took me two weeks more of my holiday before I could walk along the beach without feeling dizzy. But on the drive back to Bavaria, the dizziness returned. We only narrowly avoided an accident because I was sitting behind the wheel, thinking I was all right. At the last moment, I managed to bring the car to a halt on the hard shoulder. My wife drove us the rest of the way. Things didn't get any better at home either. I lay in bed, dizzy and weak. I couldn't even read my e-mails without breaking out in a sweat and fainting.

After a further two weeks with no noticeable improvement in my condition, I was convinced that I was seriously ill. The most plausible explanation I could think of was a brain tumour. My symptoms were the closest match; it couldn't just be sunstroke. But I was reluctant to accept the diagnosis and decided to give myself another week. Nothing changed in this week either. I was now certain that I had a tumour. There was no point in ignoring the problem any more. I made an appointment for a brain scan the next day.

I couldn't sleep the night before the examination. A thought occurred to me: if I really did have a brain tumour and my neighbour had the gift of healing with Healing Voices, but didn't trust himself to do it out of false modesty, that would be a great pity for me. I thought "too bad". I don't know why the words formed in English rather than German that night. I still don't know today.

At four o'clock in the morning, a realisation dawned. Perhaps I had no right to withhold this gift from my patients, or indeed the whole world. I made a deal with the universe. "If the examination tomorrow turns out well," I said, "if I get well, then I'll go out into the world with Healing Voices, then I'll put the method right at the top of my website and treat anyone who wants to be treated with it."

The MRI was normal – no tumour nor indeed anything else. Within three days, all my symptoms had disappeared.

Since then, I have been using Healing Voices in my practice in Bad Tölz and online worldwide. Clients rest on a comfortable chair while they benefit from the remedial effect of the Healing Voices. Even if the symptom or illness is concentrated at a specific part of the body, the Healing Voices unfold their effect on all levels, harmonise the entire body and also release blockages on a mental and spiritual level. The client is treated as a whole.

With this form of application, the client does not have to do anything other than open up to the healing energies and welcome them in.

A conscious understanding on the part of the client as to why he or she is ill, where his or her illness comes from, is not necessary in this treatment setting. It's a bit like when the doctor gives you an injection. You lie there, the doctor or shaman does something and afterwards you feel better. However, this comparison is flawed, because the injection works on the physical level in isolation, whereas the shamanic healing energies work on all levels of the client, on the body, the soul and the mind.

This type of energy healing often leads to an alleviation of symptoms and makes a significant contribution to complete healing. But this is not always enough. There are symptoms, illnesses and other life disorders where the client's consciousness plays an important, sometimes central role in the healing process. In this case, the client must understand where the illness comes from, where the real energetic cause of the problem is.

In these cases, I first do a symptom constellation. Only when the energetic cause – usually an unresolved trauma – has been discovered and all the positions involved have been set up in the constellation do the Healing Voices come into play, but then all the more powerfully. The client discovers what the shamanic energies, which work through Healing Voices, do and with whom.

**The origin**

I learnt everything I know about Healing Voices and their enormous healing energies by making myself available as a medium, as an intermediary. Even now, I am still learning more with every passing day.

However, I cannot give you any precise information about the origin of the shamanic-energetic healing powers that are at work in Healing Voices. As with the question of where life comes from, the question of the origin of Healing Voices cannot ultimately be answered. This is because shamanic healing powers are part of life, part of the general life energy and therefore also part of human nature, which is closely connected to the universal life force. As with life itself, Healing Voices simply exist. As with life, they are much greater than the human being. The human being lives, but does not make life. The human being experiences healing, but does not do the healing.

Ever since humans have existed, they have sought to explore the origins of life. They want to understand life. But the question of the origin of life has not yet been answered and will probably remain unanswered in the future.

Nevertheless, we can learn something about life and its healing powers, because life and also the energetic healing powers can be recognised as something effective and therefore existent through their effects and phenomena. The phenomena of life manifest themselves every day. On the basis of our own personal experience, it would never cross our mind that life does not exist, because we experience its effects every minute.

The phenomena of Healing Voices can also be experienced in their effects, namely in their healing effects. If a pain disappears or an illness heals after a Healing Voices treatment, then I can draw conclusions about the existence of the healing powers of Healing Voices. When you have experienced this thousands of times over decades, you could no longer conceive that Healing Voices did not exist.

They exist and surround us at all times. Just as we can enjoy life, even though we still do not know the origin of life, we can also enjoy the benefits of shamanic healing without having to understand where exactly the origin of these powerful healing forces lies.

Of course, the phenomenon of Healing Voices will continue to be researched. I do nothing else when I invite them in every day for my clients. This research makes perfect sense, even if it is not to be expected that the origin of these forces can be scientifically revealed. But when Healing Voices are used, there is a flow of information about the qualities they possess, about what exactly they do with the psychic energies in the field, about what they are connected to and what they are not connected to, about whether there are different types of healing powers, about how everything interacts and, above all, about the effects that are possible and to be expected through shamanic healing.

This is precisely what I am reporting on in this book. But first let us take a look at the technique. What exactly does a medium do so that Healing Voices can begin their healing work?

### The medium

When I work as a medium, I completely cast off my ego. I have acquired the ability to do this over decades on a long professional path under the tutelage of many teachers, a path that was sometimes crisis-ridden, and sometimes beset by extremely painful personal experiences. Shedding the ego is one of the hardest lessons to learn on the path of personal development if you want to progress along the path of maturity. This applies to everyone, no matter what they do for a living. Life itself sets us this task. It is a challenge that not all people accept. Those who consciously set out on this path have a sometimes hard, but always extremely fascinating and exciting journey ahead of them, which ultimately leads to the joy of existence. As always, there is no guarantee of success in the important endeavours of life. The journey is the destination.

However, this is not enough for an individual who wants to be available as a medium for shamanic healing energies. The goal of 'egolessness' must be achieved so that the individual's own channel is pure enough to allow the healing energies of Healing Voices to pass through unfiltered and unaltered.

Even if you remain a completely normal person in everyday life and may continue to have wishes and fears, as a medium you shed all fears and ideas as soon as you issue the invitation to the shamanic healing powers.

But what is this thing, this ego, that you have to cast off in the course of training to become a Healing Voices healer?

## The ego

It is that part of a person that feels separate from other people, basically from the whole world. The ego, the formation of the ability to recognise and experience oneself in separation from others, is an important part of human development. A child that initially feels itself in unity with its mother develops a sense of self in the first years of its life by experiencing itself as separate from its parents and siblings. You know that this time has come when the child utters the word "I" for the first time.

Depending on the cultural environment, the sense of self is more or less expanded on into adulthood, while the sense of community, the sense of unity, the awareness that one is also part of a community and a greater whole, decreases.

When the sense of I/me/mine becomes too strong, we speak of the 'ego principle', in which one's own self becomes more important than the community. I want, I need, I want, e.g. love, security, influence, money, power. We feel separated and see the other person as an enemy against whom we have to assert ourselves. Behind this is the fear that the small human ego has of dissolution, of extinction, of death.

In the personal sphere, an exaggerated ego principle leads to separation from fellow human beings. Egotistical people are not welcome. They become lonely and, in extreme cases, embittered.

In the collective, social sphere, an exaggerated ego principle leads to the exploitation of other people (get-rich-quick mentality), the exploitation of nature (earth as the dominion of mankind), the oppression of minorities (only we have the right to be here) and to war and destruction (attack or be attacked). Strength, assertiveness and ruthlessness dominate the economic and political fields.

In the course of human life, however, there is an inner counterforce that is inherent in human development from the very beginning. In this counterforce, the realisation grows in us that, although we are each an independent personality, we are at the same time connected on a deep level with everyone and everything and are basically in an inseparable unity with everything. This is the path that leads us to wisdom.

Progressing along the path of wisdom, we lose our fear of death and extinction because we feel safe and secure in the greater whole at all times. We no longer see only our own self, but also the community, we go along with the greater whole without judging it and place our self and our actions at the service of others. The 'I' becomes the 'we', from which no one is excluded.

Our own will becomes unimportant, personal influence secondary, any arrogance unthinkable. We see ourselves as part of life on this earth, part of humanity, part of everything that exists. This also means surrendering control over events and developing trust in the greater whole.

While the child and the young person find themselves in the separation of their ego, the maturing person finds themselves in the acceptance of their connections to the entire world. The ego is absorbed into the greater whole. We recognise ourselves in unity and now know who we really are.

All complacency falls away, every self-centred desire dissolves. We are at peace with ourselves, stand joyfully and powerfully in the service of the community, love life and our fellow human beings.

On a collective level, the antagonism ends. Exploitation, marginalisation, wars and environmental destruction become a thing of the past. To achieve this, large sections of humanity would have to renounce the ego principle and see themselves as part of the greater system that is our planet. Obviously, this is still a dream of the future. Humanity is still in the youthful boorish phase, in which people selfishly seize everything just because they can, are carried away by their own possibilities and do not yet have the wisdom to consider the consequences for themselves and others and make them the basis of their actions.

On a personal level, there is no need to wait for others to realise or for humanity as a whole to become wise. Each person can progress on their personal path of wisdom and maturity according to their own strength and ability.

What does this mean in the context of this book?

The ego interferes with the work of every psychotherapist, every constellator and every shamanic healer in two ways:

## The blinkers of arrogance

If, because of an inflated ego and the fundamental arrogance that stems from it, you believe that you know how everything is connected from the outset because of your experience and training, you won't see the truth. You will be blind to the reality. As a constellator you won't see the thread that leads to the original trauma in the client's energy field.

An inflated ego makes working as a medium for Healing Voices completely impossible because, as a human being, you don't know what the healing energies that work through Healing Voices will do from one moment to the next and why. The idea that you already know what will happen in the next moment or what Healing Voices should do next is presumptuous and immediately causes the flow of healing energy to dry up.

As a medium, you follow the movements and sounds in every second without judging anything, without speeding anything up, slowing anything down, directing, omitting or adding anything. You are a pure instrument, a pure channel, nothing else. If you want to be more because your ego becomes inflated ("What a great guy I am!"), you will fall out of your role. Then, instantly, nothing works anymore.

During a Healing Voices treatment, the medium's ego is put to the test every second. As soon as it comes to the fore, the movement stops, the sounds become false and inappropriate. The magic is broken. When the ego disappears because the medium remembers his/her proper place in the universe, the healing continues.

One of the most important elements of training students to become a Healing Voices practitioner is to create a framework in which they can get to know their ego and consciously cast it off. This is a big and important step for every person. In this way, participants in the training programme will experience a boost in their own personal development. This has an impact on their entire life. Because when your ego becomes smaller, your own soul releases powerful energies that lead to a rich and fulfilling life.

### False modesty

A special trick played by the ego is to deny the greater whole by sabotaging, by failing to recognise and acknowledge the power and weight which flows to us from the greater whole and to which we are entitled. We refuse to take our proper place in the world, where our inherent and intended possibilities and abilities could unfold freely.

This leads to false modesty, in which we fail to stand by our own strength and mission, in which we even actively reject it by hiding our own light under a bushel and saying thing like "That's too big for me", "I'm not that important", "I don't belong there", "I can't do it", "I'm not going to do it", "I'm too weak, too unimportant" etc.

When someone refuses to take his or her proper place, however, the greater whole becomes severely disrupted and manifests itself in the recipient with symptoms, illnesses and, in extreme cases, death. Not accepting your own greatness makes you ill!

Many shamans have experienced this when they initially did not follow the inner call and refused to follow the greater whole. They were often led back to their path by a serious illness.

I too experienced this when I refused to work with Healing Voices for years. Through a serious and protracted health disorder, I was 'forged' into a willingness to agree to my calling in this area.

This effect is also familiar with other life tasks that are assigned to you by the greater whole. Many people unconsciously suffer from their refusal to follow a professional path or an inner calling that beckons.

Recognising false modesty, standing by your inner and outer greatness and following your calling is sometimes difficult. Even if you already understand yourself as part of the greater whole, this basic understanding on an intellectual level is sometimes not enough. This is because development is often severely disrupted or made impossible by unconscious blockages.

These blockages can come from the social milieu in which you grew up. It is sometimes difficult to leave your social class ("Cobbler, stick to thy last!") and be successful in your own career because of an unconscious solidarity with your family of origin. Or a former family member has been prevented by fate, war or death from realising their professional dreams; through solidarity with your own family, you yourself are blocked.

People who are called to be healers often have an additional blockage. It can be traced back to an unresolved trauma in a previous life. A typical example is the torture and murder by the Catholic Inquisition in the Middle Ages of women and men who practised shamanic healing or applied traditional herbal knowledge, using the knowledge of the old matriarchal religions. The fear of being murdered again because of this activity as a healer can leap across the boundary to the present life and typically emerges at the moment when such a person wants to show his or her healing abilities in public, e.g. at a lecture, on the internet or in social networks. The result is unconscious paralysis. The potential healer simply doesn't make any progress or doesn't even start.

The good news is that these blockages can be released with a symptom constellation in combination with Healing Voices.

In the course of training to become a Healing Voices practitioner, the release of such blockages or similar is an important step enabling students to become free and grow into their full power and greatness.

Collective social influences can also elicit false modesty. In social systems in which a few powerful people seek to preserve their power by keeping the majority of their subjects (or electorate) weak and powerless, healthy self-confidence cannot develop in the disadvantaged sections of the population. Religious dogmas, which tell the ordinary people that they are basically small, unworthy sinners, also play an important role.

Breaking out of these socially prescribed moulds is a major task. Here too, constellations in their collective form can support liberation on a personal level. In collective constellations, the greatest healing effect also comes from Healing Voices!

### Fear as a stumbling block

Along with arrogance and false modesty, fear is the biggest stumbling block encountered by a potential medium for Healing Voices.

Two different types of fear stand out here:

On the one hand, the fundamental fear felt by the ego – the human ego that thinks itself separate – of dissolving, of being defenceless and helpless, of being completely unimportant and lost in the big, hostile universe. We believe that we will not be able to achieve the goals we have set ourselves – our planned career, our own house, car, boat – if we don't assert ourselves, if we don't know where we are going, if we don't propel ourselves into the future with the aid of our own magnificence.

As a medium for Healing Voices, you have to admit to yourself every second that you don't know where it goes from here, you don't know what will happen next, you have no idea how exactly Healing Voices heal. You have to leave it to the greater whole, to the shamanic-energetic healing forces that are part of this greater whole.

The ego only interferes here. Surrendering the ego means agreeing that, as a human being, you are in a very safe place in the game of the universe, that you will always have what you need, including on the material level, and that you are surrounded by great supportive forces and strong shamanic healing powers that help you and protect you from harm. If you adopt this inner attitude, there is no reason for fear. You are safe at all times.

On the other hand, fears that lurk unrecognised in the shadow areas of your own energy field play an important role. These fears often go back to unresolved, fear-inducing traumas in the family system, in your own personal experience in this present life or to an unresolved trauma from a previous incarnation.

Fears that lie encapsulated in the unconscious can be activated by external events in a matter of seconds. The experience of making yourself available as a medium for Healing Voices is a field in which such external events occur regularly.

In symptom constellations, the shamanic-energetic healing energies are often confronted by aggression and negative energies. In particular, perpetrators who are occupied by negative energy try to defend themselves against the healing forces. Sometimes there is conflict between positive and negative energies. It is true that the healing, light-filled side is always somewhat stronger than the destructive, dark side. However, the ability to endure the flow of strong healing energies, which are necessary to free the energy field of a constellation from the energy of the perpetrator, requires a channel that is free of fear. If your own unconscious fears exist and are provoked in this situation, you will lose contact with the healing powers at that moment. Under certain circumstances, this can be dangerous for the medium, because in such a situation burdened souls can attach themselves energetically to the medium.

I recall the case of an alternative practitioner who was convinced that she could free a client of a negative force that had taken spiritual possession of him, although she had neither the necessary training nor the personal maturity and strength.

In the weeks that followed, the practitioner had three major accidents, which she, like the other road users, miraculously survived with minor injuries. The symptom constellation revealed that the negative force that was possessing the client had energetically leapt across and attached itself to the healer and had begun to endanger her health and her life. With the help of Healing Voices, it was possible to free her from the negative force.

In order to avoid such situations and to protect yourself as a healer, it is an important and necessary part of training to bring light into the darkness of your own shadow areas and to actively identify and dissipate the fears that lie there.

The type of constellation I have developed for this is called a 'Shadow Constellation'. You do not wait until an anxiety symptom indicates that a shadow area is ripe for inspection and resolution. Instead, you proactively look for these areas in the shadow constellation in order to take preventive measures and pre-empt an unpleasant or potentially dangerous situation in a Healing Voices treatment that the student will later carry out.

## Basic settings for Healing Voices

There are three different settings in which Healing Voices are used.

1. ### Healing Voices without Symptom Constellation

   The client lies passively on a couch. The therapist invites the shamanic healing energies and carries out the Healing Voices treatment. The treatment takes about 20 to 30 minutes.

   It is sufficient if the illness, symptom or problem is named in the introductory conversation. The client opens up to the shamanic healing powers without having to do anything themselves. It is very similar to a doctor giving an injection. The client does not know how it all works. The doctor or therapist does something and afterwards the client is better. The client learns nothing about the energetic background, where the problem comes from or why it occurs. Nevertheless, a remedial change comes about. This type of Healing Voices treatment can be carried out in the treatment room or online. The effect is just as strong online as in the face-to-face situation in the practitioner's treatment room. For some symptoms, illnesses or problems, a Healing Voices treatment alone is not sufficient for complete healing. In these cases, I recommend combining Healing Voices with a symptom constellation.

2. ### Healing Voices in combination with a symptom constellation

   In this setting, a symptom constellation is carried out before the Healing Voices are applied. This can take place in a therapy group or in individual treatment. The therapy group, as well as the individual treatment, can take place in person or online.

The symptom constellation reveals the energetic cause of the problem, symptom or illness. The client thus learns where the original trauma lies that has led to the current problem. This expands the client's consciousness. The realisation of how everything is connected in the background already has a healing effect. The force behind the problem usually diminishes at this point.

For deeper healing, however, further healing movements in the client's energy field are necessary, which can only be carried out by Healing Voices. While Healing Voices are active with the help of the medium, you can see in the constellation which people and positions they are working with.

The expanded consciousness of the client and the shamanic healing powers, which work in the invisible energy fields of all those involved, operate together in this setting, which usually leads to a much deeper healing experience. This is because the client now also understands how everything is connected and experiences how the burden is released. The message of the symptom is delivered and accepted. The deeper meaning of the symptom is thus fulfilled. The symptom can now withdraw.

3. **Healing Voices in a collective constellation**

Healing Voices can also be used in collective constellations to create a deeper healing experience for all participants. In principle, the process is very similar to a personal symptom constellation. However, the healing effects naturally affect more people – ideally the entire collective, society or nation.

Healing Voices can also be used successfully on animals and plants. The results of the Healing Voices treatments I have carried out for animals and plants so far are very encouraging. However, there is still a lot of research to be done in this area.

## The preparation of the clients

Every person who participates in a Healing Voices treatment needs to be prepared for what is to come. A safe environment is required so that the client or alternatively the group members, if the treatment takes place in a group, feel comfortable.

That is why I always give a detailed introduction, after which the clients know that the shamanic-energetic healing energies that work in Healing Voices surround us at all times, that they are strong and often ready to help us. However, they cannot become active on their own, as two important prerequisites must be met.

Firstly, the client has to say 'yes' and mean it. Healing Voices cannot do anything without the client's full consent, because they obviously respect the free will of us humans.

Secondly, the shamanic healing powers need a person who is able and willing to act as a channel, as a medium for them.

I make myself available for the function of the medium in the settings described above. In the constellation setting, I introduce a new position, which I define as the 'Position of the Healers'. I then place myself in this position as a representative and invite the shamanic-energetic healing energies to perform healing action in the client's systemic field.

Part of the introduction is also to give an outlook on what can happen in the constellation after the invitation has been extended to the healing forces. The clients should be prepared for the fact that healing takes place with gestures, sounds and words or even sentences from archaic languages. They should know that the voices can become very loud and aggressive when working in victim-perpetrator fields. The clients need to know that they do not have to be afraid, even in these phases of healing, and that they are in a safe environment. I guarantee this before every Healing Voices treatment. Even though I work as a medium, I am not in a trance but very consciously present and can also step out of the healer's position at any time if necessary.

I also prepare the clients for the fact that the Healing Voices often work with the souls of the victims after the loud and aggressive phase. In this phase you can sometimes hear lamenting and grieving sounds. The deeper meaning is obviously to allow the grief, which is always present somewhere in perpetrator-victim fields, to flow.

After that, the Healing Voices become softer and more melodic. In this phase, they often come into the client's immediate environment to provide energetic support to him or her in releasing any remaining burdensome energy.

The client should be informed about all of this before the shamanic healing begins.

Because astonishing things often happen during a Healing Voices treatment that go beyond the scope of what has been experienced so far, I also prepare the clients for this by telling them that they should not be surprised about anything during the session, because very unusual things can happen in a shamanic healing. I always repeat at this point that everyone present is safe.

If the shamanic healing takes place in a therapy group, I also inform all group members present about another amazing phenomenon of Healing Voices, namely that they do not confine themselves to the set framework of a client's personal symptom constellation, but often also offer their healing powers to the 'watching' participants in the group. It is therefore possible that group participants who are not involved in the constellation can also have physical and emotional healing experiences on a very personal level. Every participant should be informed about this. The group participants themselves decide whether or not to open themselves up to such a healing experience. As I said, Healing Voices respect people's free will. If someone really only wants to be a spectator and a witness to what is happening, it suffices to make that inner decision and distance him or herself.

Nevertheless, a Healing Voices treatment is always a special experience for all those present. Everyone present knows that healing energies are conveyed through the gestures, voices and chants.

### The invitation

At the beginning there is always an invitation that I extend to the shamanic-energetic energies, regardless of whether it is a pure Healing Voices treatment without a constellation or a Healing Voices session as part of a symptom constellation.

Because I often have the impression during my work as a medium with Healing Voices that different healing and sound qualities are used, which are conveyed by different, personified qualities and entities, I choose the personified form 'Healers' as the form of address in the invitation. Since I basically do not know who will respond to my invitation and from which geographical areas or historical eras the healing entities originate, I choose the following invitation formula:

**"I invite you, Healers of all times, both male and female, to heal in the client's system on all levels, if you are willing and able."**

When you extend the above invitation, you must always realise anew that you are not the healer yourself, but that it is the Healers from the healing field who carry out the healing. That is why the

Healers themselves decide whether they do something or not and whether the situation is suitable for such action.

It happened to me at the beginning that I issued the invitation in a situation in which the application of shamanic healing powers was obviously not appropriate. In these cases, the Healers did not use my channel. There was no impulse, no movement, no sound, nothing.

In retrospect I always understood why it wasn't the right time or the right situation. Usually, my ego wanted too much or the symptom constellation was missing a person who was necessary to understand the unresolved trauma.

But if the situation is right, then the shamanic healing begins immediately after I have extended the invitation.

## The implementation

The basis for a successful Healing Voices treatment is that the medium is aware of his or her role and function as a pure tool. I make myself available for every second of the healing. As long as it lasts – often 10 to 20 minutes – I lend Healing Voices my body for gestures and my voice for sounds. I am only a medium and allow everything else to happen without intervening. I follow the impulses in every millisecond, without judgement, without slowing anything down and without amplifying anything. I follow the movement impulses millimetre by millimetre. I never know how a movement will continue, where it will lead and where it will end. Gestures are often formed with hands and arms as the Healers move step by step through the constellation. Sometimes they touch someone, work with their hands in the aura or energetically in a person's body. If necessary, they draw out burdensome energies from the client or another person in the field of the constellation. You never know what will happen from one moment to the next.

It's the same with the sounds. First there is a brief silence. I let go of my voice. Then a sound, then the next. Sometimes I hear the next sound even before it leaves my throat. Sometimes my mouth forms words or even sentences that I don't understand. Because they obviously come from ancient, archaic languages. Sometimes the words and sentences remind me of Japanese, Chinese, Russian, French or other languages. The Healers rarely give lengthy 'speeches' or 'talks'.

You can't understand the archaic words with your mind, but you can with your heart. Intuitively, you realise who they are addressed to and what they mean in the context.

During a Healing Voices treatment, it remains a challenge for the medium to put aside his or her ego, the small and petty human ego, and to stop it taking the lead at any time. I remember a situation in a therapy seminar in England in which I moved through the constellation during Healing Voices as a medium and group leader at the same time, singing melodies and rolling on the floor. I was briefly struck by the thought of what I, a qualified doctor of medicine, was actually doing, rolling across the floor and singing to heal an illness. What would the chief physicians, under whom I had worked for many years as a junior doctor, say if they saw me now?

It was only a brief moment. I already had enough experience with shamanic healings not to become insecure at this point. I let my ego go again and moved into the safety of my greater self, which knows that it is connected to everything, safe and secure in the cosmos from which Healing Voices are generated.

### Experience and the present moment

Before I describe the various phases in which a Healing Voices treatment takes place, I would like to emphasise that experience plays a completely subordinate role here. The dominant element is the therapist's ability to follow the impulses of the shamanic healing energies as a medium in every moment. This cannot be emphasised often enough.

### The most important thing is the ability to follow the impulses of the moment!

### Experience is secondary

The ability to follow the impulses of the moment without fear and without judgement is sufficient to carry out a Healing Voices treatment. However, it usually takes years of training to develop this ability in its pure form.

Obviously, you learn something when you make yourself available as a medium for shamanic healing energies. Over the course of time, this builds up a wealth of experience, which is certainly beneficial, but must never be allowed to impair your ability to follow the impulses of the moment. There is always a danger if you believe, based on your experience, that you already know what will or should happen next.

For teaching purposes, however, accumulated experience is helpful. It prepares students who are on the path to becoming Healing Voices therapists for what might await them during healing, but not for what actually will await them. It is also helpful to witness many examples of Healing Voices treatments in training

On the following pages I would therefore like to speak from my experience and describe the typical phases in which a Healing Voices treatment can take place, depending on the setting.

### The phases of a Healing Voices treatment

In a **Healing Voices treatment without symptom constellation,** in which the client lies on a couch and experiences the healing passively, the shamanic healing energies work in harmonising and balancing fashion in the client's energy field. Neither the client nor the therapist as medium knows what exactly is happening or on which levels Healing Voices are currently working. Sometimes the medium has the impression that burdensome energies are being drawn out of the client's body or soul. There have also been situations in which I, as a doctor, intuitively knew which organ the Healing Voices were working with and what exactly they were putting right. Sometimes energetic 'operations' are carried out. In these cases it is not necessary for the client to know about it. What is important is what happens on an energy level.

Often Healing Voices also bring positive, light-filled energies from the universe to the client, which significantly supports the healing process.

This type of Healing Voices treatment lasts around 15 to 20 minutes. Loud or aggressive sounds are rarely used. At the end of the session, there is often a harmonising phase in which the energies are balanced and smoothed out.

During a **Healing Voices treatment in a symptom constellation,** the medium, and often also the client, knows in which positions and which areas of the constellation the shamanic healing forces are currently working. There are typical phases that vary slightly depending on the individual case. Knowing these typical phases is important for all therapists who wish to make themselves available as a medium for Healing Voices. However, there is no 'instruction manual'. Every Healing Voices treatment is new and unique. Even if experience shows that some phases are repeated in multiple constellations, you should never expect to be able to draw conclusions about the next case.

### Working with perpetrators and aggression

In perpetrator-victim fields, Healing Voices work in a very powerful initial phase with the negative forces and aggression of the perpetrators. Here the medium is particularly challenged to abandon all judgement and evaluation of what is going on. The sounds coming from Healing Voices can become extremely loud and aggressive in these situations. This includes expressions of aggression such as hissing, roaring, malicious laughter and other primordial sound elements that are unfamiliar from everyday life. The sounds can be disturbing at first. However, it is important that these tonal qualities can also flow unhindered through the medium and become audible in this way. This is because it is not just about the audible sounds, but essentially about the healing energies that they convey in the invisible and inaudible realm. If a medium were to interrupt these sounds and noises, the effective healing energies that are conveyed by these sounds would also be interrupted.

As a medium, you must not become afraid at this point, otherwise you will fall out of your role as a medium. The flow of healing energies will dry up. This can also be dangerous for you as the therapist in situations where you are dealing with negative energies. Because if you become afraid, you depart from the role of the medium and therefore also leave the energy field that is protected by the Healing Voices. You become weakened. Negative psychic energies can then attach themselves to you as the therapist. The result can be depressed energies, panic or even health hazards, including the risk of accidents, which can last for weeks.

Therefore, as already emphasised, thorough training is necessary in which you as a medium can see and resolve your own fear potentials in the shadow areas of your personal energy field. Once your own shadow areas have been resolved, it is safe to work with negative energies and fields of aggression.

In your role as a medium, it is important that you develop full trust in the shamanic healing powers of Healing Voices and feel completely safe at all times. This is because perpetrator-victim fields are common in symptom constellations. On an almost daily basis in my individual therapies, I see how Healing Voices disempower the perpetrators, destroy their energy and remove them from the system. Nazi perpetrators, including Hitler, are shouted down, perpetrators of the Catholic Inquisition are disabled and destroyed, murderers and slave hunters are chased out of the system. The list of perpetrators disempowered and destroyed by Healing Voices is long. Because I work with clients from many different countries, the perpetrators whose disempowerment I have witnessed as a medium come from many cultures and countries. Because I work with unresolved traumas in past lives, they also belong to many different eras in history.

The effect of Healing Voices in this area is always the same. The perpetrators, who have entered into such a strong connection with negative energies that they cannot be separated from them through the healing, are energetically disempowered. In a constellation, the representatives of the perpetrators lie down on the floor in this phase and have the sensation that they are sinking into the ground. This category of perpetrator regularly includes mass murderers, serial killers, fanatical Nazis, war criminals of various backgrounds and many others.

Perpetrators who have entered into only a slight connection with negative energies can be separated from the negative energy by Healing Voices. Suddenly, something falls away from them, their heart opens to compassion, they become human again, suddenly see the victims and their suffering and realise what they have really done. The scales fall from their eyes. These perpetrators fall to their knees in deep remorse before the victims and weep bitterly over what they have done. This takes a long time – much longer than a constellation or a workshop. The length of time that the souls of these perpetrators remain in remorse cannot be measured in normal time.

It is important to know that the perpetrators or perpetrator organisations are only destroyed in the client's personal energy field, i.e. in the family of origin or in a particular previous incarnation. They are still active in other families, other incarnations or in society. If mass murderers such as Hitler, Catholic inquisitors and so on are disempowered in a particular family system, they are far from being disempowered in other families and in society as a whole. There, they are still energetically present and active. As a constellator, you therefore have to start again from scratch in every symptom constellation. Healing Voices also start again from the beginning. I have lost count of the number of families in which I have experienced the disempowerment of Hitler and other mass murderers. There are also countless cases in which I, as a medium in reincarnation constellations, have witnessed the disempowerment of the Catholic Church and its torturers or of pharaohs or other tyrannical rulers. The cleansing of the energy field from the perpetrators must be carried out anew in every system.

Healing Voices always work with the perpetrators first, then with the souls of the victims. In all these years, I have never experienced it being the other way round. So, there is method behind it.

## Working with the souls of the victims

An essential part of a Healing Voices treatment in a perpetrator-victim field is working with the souls of the victims or, in the case of fateful death without the involvement of perpetrators, working with the souls of those who have died before their allotted time.

Experience has shown that there are two phases: firstly, working with the grief, and secondly, releasing the affected souls from the trauma freeze.

## Working with grief

An essential element of the trauma process is blocked grief. The grief over the early death of a loved one, especially if it occurs suddenly or is the result of a violent crime, can be so overwhelming that relatives have no choice but to protect themselves from this deep pain by blocking all feelings. This can lead to a full-blown trauma of loss, in which one or more relatives close themselves off to such an extent that they will not be free of this emotional blockage for the rest of their life and will live as if frozen, like someone who is already dead inside, a dead person in a living body, no longer capable of any response.

The blockage of grief, which is often passed down through the generations to the descendants, can also cross the boundary to a later incarnation and emerge in the current life as an incomprehensible burden.

Healing Voices often mourn for the dead instead of the relatives in order to restore the flow of grief in the system. In a constellation, the medium is often observed kneeling down with the victims, weeping and mourning out loud. This stimulates the grief in the entire system and allows it to flow. The representatives of the immediate family and their descendants experience this strongly in the constellations. They also burst into tears, as the grief that has been hidden away somewhere for a long time can now also be released in them.

Any feeling that is blocked becomes a problem. When that feeling can flow, healing happens.

This phase can last several minutes in a Healing Voices treatment, depending on how many victims or deceased persons the shamanic healing energies are working with.

The wailing can sound very primordial. It can be quite a challenge for a therapist who is experiencing Healing Voices as a medium for the first time. This is because, if there is unresolved grief in the medium's unconscious, that will also be stimulated. The medium becomes sad of his own accord or even flooded with an unconscious grief from his or her own system. The medium then falls out of role, can no longer fulfil the function of the medium and is personally in need of help. The healing is interrupted at this point.

Healing Voices training therefore emphasises the importance of discovering and healing unresolved grief in the student's energy field. Most people have multiple areas of grief in their unconscious. The release of these areas is necessary in order to be able to take on the function of a medium, unencumbered by them. Lamentations, however primordial, strong and loud they may be, are then no longer a problem for the medium. The transition to the next phase is smooth and natural.

In the next phase, something absolutely amazing happens: the liberation of the souls of the victims and the deceased from the trauma freeze.

## Releasing souls from trauma

The fact that a soul can freeze in fatal trauma is central to understanding the phenomenon. As a result of trauma freeze, negative emotions are experienced again and again in an endless loop, thereby entering the energy field of the entire system and being passed down through generations or flowing into a later incarnation.

After the grief in the system has been brought into flow through shamanic healing, Healing Voices dedicate themselves to the task of liberating the souls from the trauma freeze.

This phase immediately follows the 'mourning phase' or, more precisely expressed, it emerges from the depths of grief. What can be seen to happen in the constellation is as follows:

The medium kneels down to the victims, most of whom are lying on the ground. While the mourning continues, a melody is woven into the sounds of grief, the hands make spiralling gestures and movements that lead upwards, as if slowly establishing a connection to a brighter, redeeming energy. The medium slowly stands up and helps the soul in question out of the frozen trauma with chants and movements. In the constellation, the representatives of the victims follow this movement with a slight delay. They slowly rise from the floor and straighten up while the medium is already standing upright and often opens his or her arms upwards as in a resurrection.

The awakening of the victims' souls from the trauma, the slow realisation that the atmosphere around them is changing, that the perpetrators have clearly been destroyed and disappeared, that a bright and liberating energy is increasingly surrounding them, lifting them up, opening their eyes and freeing their minds, takes several minutes and continues even while the shamanic energies working through the medium are already attending to the needs of the next victim. The liberation of the victims or those who died before their allotted time span has primordial traits, goes emotionally deep and is also shared with the people who experience the healing in the group. The liberation runs through the generations of the family and can also be clearly felt by the client, who may be the grand-daughter or great-granddaughter of the victim. The trauma is released. The energy in the entire room changes, becoming lighter and brighter.

When this liberating movement is fully developed, some victims can be seen standing upright, arms outstretched upwards, freed from suffering and pain, free from aggression or revenge. They feel wonderful and are now ready to go the way they are obviously meant to go after death, into the light.

A second reaction that victims manifest after being freed from trauma freeze is regularly seen when there have been many victims, especially in cases of genocide and mass murder. In such cases, the freed victims make eye contact with the many other victims who have also just been freed from the trauma and form a community with them again. They often stand in a large semi-circle, place their arms on each other's shoulders and make swinging body move-ments. Sometimes they also enter into a dance of joy together, while some of them stand with their arms outstretched upwards, ready to connect with the greater whole.

The liberation of the victims is also a healing process for the client, because at this moment he or she is also freed from his or her energetic burden. When the ancestors affected by the trauma emerge from it, there is no longer any reason to carry their burden. It simply no longer makes sense. The client can now let go of the energetic burden more easily.

However, shamanic healing is not yet complete at this point. It is still in full swing, because there is still more to do. Now that the victims have been freed from the trauma freeze, many things be-come possible that were previously impossible.

## Liberating mourners from shutdown

Even if the victims are freed from the trauma freeze, the grieving immediate family are often not. This is because the loss may itself have become a trauma. Some immediate family members are stuck in this trauma of loss. They are still in the trauma freeze of their grief. They too sometimes need the healing impulses of Healing Voices. As with the victims, the shamanic healing powers make intimate contact with the souls of the mourners and ease them out of their depression with healing chants and gestures, slowly opening their eyes to the fact that the lost loved one is already standing close to them, upright and freed from their trauma.

The representatives of the mourners often report that they first sense their loved ones, then see them as if through a fog, disbelieving at first, only to see more clearly and realise that it is reality after all, actual reality. Then something happens that is deeply healing for everyone involved and for the entire system: the person who is grieving and the deceased loved one feel an attraction that is mixed with love and joy. A joyful, intimate connection comes about between souls who have been separated by fate for so long.

## Connection of separated souls

The separation of people deeply connected through love is the strongest disturbance in the system that can be imagined. It is the greatest suffering from which later generations cannot escape, even if they have never heard of the ancestors concerned and of their fate.

Healing happens when the connection between separated souls is re-established. Right from the start, Healing Voices work to revitalise severed connections. Examples of this are as follows: lovers who have been separated by illness, accident, murder or war and find each other again on a spiritual-energetic level through Healing

Voices; a great-grandmother who regains access to the souls of her five children who died as babies, a woman who reconnects with the soul of an aborted or miscarried child; a son who reconnects with his father, whom he found dead at the age of eight after the father had committed suicide. The list of examples is endless.

The reuniting of two souls who belong together happens as if by magic during a Healing Voices treatment. Sometimes the shamanic energies actively support this development in the energy field of the person concerned. In the constellation, the medium can be seen making connecting gestures between the two people. These gestures sometimes seem like multiple infinity loops, but they are never the same; they are slightly different each time, like the waves on the beach. They also resemble each other and yet each wave is unique.

Incidentally, the image of waves on the beach is a very apt analogy for the movements of a medium during a Healing Voices sequence. Just as the wave unquestioningly yields and moulds itself to the forces of the infinite ocean, the medium also unquestioningly yields to the forces from the depths of the universe, from which the gestures and sounds of the shamanic healing powers are born.

In the constellation, the representatives of those affected are seen embracing each other and standing together in joy and love. This is a healing image for the client. Sometimes it is a loving couple standing together, sometimes it is a whole family with parents and several children.

This image of loving harmony also connects something in the client's soul. It becomes complete and whole. Suddenly love and joy in their full primordial dimension are also possible in the client's life.

## Work in the personal energy field

Before I work with Healing Voices in a constellation, the client in person takes their place. The representative of the client leaves the role and sits down on his or her chair

As a result, the client experiences the healing effect of the Healing Voices live in his or her own body and soul. This is particularly impressive when Healing Voices work directly in the client's energy field. This happens regularly, especially with physical illnesses and symptoms, but also with emotional burdens such as depression, anxiety and psychosis.

Healing Voices sometimes draw a burdensome energy out of the client's body and expel disturbing energies from the brain, heart, liver or other organs. Sometimes they perform energetic operations on tumours or joint and bone inflammations.

On a physical level, the body cells need a few days or weeks to adjust to the new, healed, energetic situation. Relief can come soon, but it takes some time for full healing.

## Integration of a lost soul part

The therapy of a personal trauma, whether in the current or a previous incarnation, is essentially about reintroducing a part of the soul that is frozen in the trauma to the client so that he or she can consciously and actively integrate it.

Special psychotherapeutic methods such as guided fantasy journeys are used for this purpose. However, in the case of severe traumas or a trauma in a previous incarnation, these methods are insufficient or even contraindicated in order to avoid re-traumatisation.

In such cases, I invite the shamanic energies of Healing Voices to release the soul part from the trauma field and guide it to the client (more on this in the chapter 'The therapeutic procedure in detail' starting on page 153).

The method by which the shamanic healing powers carry out the integration of a lost soul part is impressive. In the constellation, the medium can be seen releasing the soul part from the trauma and slowly and gently guiding it towards the client. The tones and chants become higher and softer. When the soul part has reached the client, the shamanic healing powers connect the soul part energetically with the client. They make undulating or spiralling movements with their hands in the client's energy field and accompany the process of merging with chants and melodies, sometimes also with primordial, empowering words.

## Harmonisation of the entire field

In the final phase of a Healing Voices treatment, the shamanic healing powers harmonise and smooth the entire energy field of the constellated system. Exactly how this happens varies from case to case; it is never the same. The healers often go through the constellation field step by step several times and make balancing movements with their hands. The sounds become more harmonious and softer. Finally, they fade away.

## Energetic preparation of the future

Sometimes the shamanic healing powers of Healing Voices prepare the future. This happens in the final phase of the healing session. The Healers may open a door to the outside, sometimes even step outside (e.g. onto the balcony, the terrace, the garden) and prepare the future field energetically for the client. Sometimes the client can already take a few steps towards the future in the constellation. In other cases, the integration of the healed situation still needs time. In such circumstances, the future is still a long way off. The client will take the first steps towards freedom and the wide-open field of the future later. But the Healers are already preparing the field, are sometimes already far away over the horizon.

### The conclusion of a shamanic healing session

It is not the medium who determines when the shamanic healing is finished, but the shamanic healing energies. As a medium, your task at this point is to follow the sound or movement impulses for as long as they last. It has happened to me a few times that I have broken off a healing before the time was up because I thought it must surely be enough. But the representatives in the constellation were only able to report a partial improvement; the victims in particular had got stuck somewhere on the way to liberation from the trauma freeze.

I had no choice but to step into the position of the Healing Voices once again as a medium. In these cases, the shamanic healing continued for several minutes until the souls of the victims had experienced full liberation and were standing upright with their arms outstretched upwards, feeling completely at ease.

There are no instructions as to how exactly the medium will sense the end of the healing. Here, too, the medium must follow the impulses of the moment. What you often see, however, is that the sounds become quieter, the breathing slower and the atmosphere becomes peaceful. Sometimes, the Healing Voices are still in the centre of the constellation field, sometimes they retreat to the edge or are already in the far distance of the future.

### Reading the effect in the constellation

At the end of the shamanic healing, I read the effect on the state of mind of the client and the representatives in the constellation. If the constellation takes place in a group, I ask each representative and, of course, the client how they are feeling now.

If the constellation takes place in an individual setting, which is often the case, then I, as the representative, go back to each position to register the state of mind of the person concerned. If there is a perpetrator-victim field, I start with the perpetrators, then go to the victims and then step into the remaining positions.

It is important that the client recognises the changes through Healing Voices in the constellation so that he or she can take this image away and remember it later.

## Healing Voices in a collective constellation

Collective constellations deal with major social issues that affect many people, such as war and peace, economic crises, the coronavirus pandemic, the environmental crisis, the marginalisation of minorities, social unrest, increased violence, racism, the dysfunctional relationship between women and men worldwide and much more besides.

Why is there a chapter on collective constellations in a book on energy medicine? What does medicine have to do with social problems or the fraught relationship between nations? The answer is that collective problems can and regularly do affect the health of individuals. Wars, understood as a disease of nations, also kill otherwise healthy people. The wrong policy decisions on epidemics jeopardise the health of millions. Economic depression leads to an increased suicide rate. Exploitation and political corruption are fuelling hunger and deprivation in many countries, leading to numerous diseases and early deaths. There are thousands of examples that show the close connection between social grievances, international crises and undesirable developments with health impairments on a very personal level.

Collective constellations that find good solutions to collective problems can therefore also be seen as part of medical action that is aimed at prevention and healing across a broad base. As with personal problems and with collective issues, systemic constellations also offer the opportunity to shine a light on the true, hidden background of a disorder and to make this information accessible to many people. At the same time, the collective constellation offers an ideal field for the shamanic healing powers of Healing Voices. People who are present when healing takes place in a collective constellation, or later watch a video recording, experience amazing healing phenomena. They feel calmer, lose their fear and feel hope again.

It is a special experience to see Healing Voices at work in a collective constellation with ninety or more positions and to be touched by the effects and healing developments. To date (2024), five large collective constellations led by me have been recorded on video and are available to the world community free of charge. You can find them on my homepage under the menu item 'Collective Constellations'.

https://www.dr-rauscher.de/en/kollektive-aufstellung

## The therapeutic procedure in detail

The procedure in a symptom constellation depends on the energetic cause that led to the problem, symptom or illness. The shamanic healing at the end of the constellation also adapts to the respective situation.

There are certain procedures that have proven successful. In this chapter, I will describe the typical procedure and the most important treatment principles in detail. At this point, however, it is important to emphasise once again that there are no user instructions for either symptom constellations or Healing Voices. Everything always develops from the moment. However, in order to be able to follow the signs of the moment better, there are key points that help us see and understand the information flowing in at that moment and the possible healing interventions in context.

These cornerstones and basic principles differ depending on which of the four major background areas the unresolved trauma occurred in:

1. Personal trauma in an individual's current life (childhood, adolescence, adulthood)
2. Personal trauma in a previous incarnation
3. Trauma in the present family
4. Trauma in a previous generation of the family of origin

### 1. Personal trauma in a current life

**Therapeutic intervention:**
Reunion with a lost or abandoned part of the soul.

The therapy of a personal trauma, whether in the current or a previous incarnation, is essentially about reintroducing the part of the soul that is frozen in the trauma to the client so that he or she can consciously integrate it.

The technique and methodology used depends on whether it is a personal trauma in the client's current life (childhood, adolescence, adulthood) or a trauma in a previous life.

In the case of an unresolved **trauma in the present life,** a part of the soul is usually frozen in the traumatic situation. Even years and decades later, this part of the soul is still in trauma shutdown. It is missing in the person concerned. That individual feels incomplete. A strength or a quality is missing. For healing to take place, the lost or frozen part of the soul must be retrieved from the past.

In order to determine whether the problem or illness the client presents with can be traced back to an unresolved trauma in his or her current life, the four-column test is carried out in the symptom constellation (see also page 100). If it is found to concern a personal trauma in the current life, I set the original trauma (not yet named) up as a new position. The constellation is then expanded to include the most important personal traumas that the client remembers. Which of the named traumas is actually the original one emerges from the constellation. As a rule, the trauma that is being sought positions itself alongside the original trauma and merges with it. If none of the named traumas shows a clear connection to the original trauma, the therapist must look further and also consider traumas that are not remembered, such as birth traumas or intrauterine traumas.

The list of possible traumas is long. It can be birth trauma, early separation or loss trauma, sexual abuse, rape, an accident, kidnapping and much more. There are countless examples.

Once the relevant trauma has been identified, the next step is to set up a part of the client's soul that may still be stuck or frozen in the trauma. As a rule, the constellation indicates the existence of this part of the soul. In the case of sexual abuse, for example, this part of the soul often feels like a child in danger.

The next step is for the client to reconnect with this part of the soul. There are two methods that complement each other:

- The therapeutically guided fantasy journey to the place and time of the trauma
- The support of shamanic healing powers (Healing Voices)

### The therapeutically guided fantasy journey
(not suitable for children and teenagers)

Depending on the type and severity of the trauma, I take the client on a guided fantasy journey back through time and to the place of the incident. The aim is to complete the soul, to make the person whole so that nothing is missing. Three things are important here:

- The client makes this journey as the adult person he or she is today.
- If there is a perpetrator, his or her energy must have already left the scene of the incident so that re-traumatisation does not occur during the fantasy journey.
- The therapist accompanies the client on the entire journey.

In the fantasy journey, I take the client back to the traumatic situation in a protected setting. In order to avoid re-traumatisation, it is important that the client makes this journey as an adult and in their adult energy. As a therapist, I accompany the client and make the setting safe.

After arriving at the place and time of the trauma, the client makes contact with his or her soul part, perhaps putting an arm

155

around it and speaking to it. The client says, for example: "We survived. Life has gone on. We have survived."

The client then walks away from the site of the trauma with the soul part and carries it through his or her life in fast motion. The client continues to speak sentences to his or her soul part, using words such as: "We survived. Now we are together again. Nothing can separate us now. I'll take care of you now."

Back in the present, I guide the client through the important ritual of reunification which I have called the 'bowl ritual':

The client forms a bowl with both hands in which the soul part is located energetically. I encourage the client to allow the soul part to sink slowly into him or herself. The client allows the soul part to move inside to where it wants to go. The hands move very slowly towards the chest or another part of the body.

The soul part knows exactly where it wants to go. It goes to the place from which it has been missing. It has been missing in every cell of the body, in every part of the soul and in every part of the client's aura. The reunion is a passive process, an acceptance and perception of where the soul part is at the moment. As it continues to expand in the client's body, it also remains in the parts where it was initially. Clients have a fine perception of where the soul part is currently moving. They perceive where this union, this becoming whole, is taking place in the body. It often begins in the chest, can then shift to the abdomen, the legs, then back to the shoulders, arms, neck and head. Later, the soul part can also move into the aura. Sometimes, invisible antennae are even formed, projecting into the wider environment, connecting the person with their surroundings and ultimately with the entire universe.

Even during the initial phase, which only lasts a few minutes, clients become aware of a pleasant, peaceful and relaxed feeling spreading through them. Movement impulses and gestures often arise in the body during this phase. Arms spread out, the hips and the whole person start to move in a gently swinging motion.

Sometimes, muscle tension that has been present for a long time becomes eased. The result is a revitalisation of the whole body. Typically, the spine straightens as if by itself.

On a spiritual level, the same happens in a corresponding form. The mood brightens, inner peace sets in. The shadows of the past trauma dissolve. In the constellation, the representative of the trauma typically lies down on the floor, has the feeling of losing all strength and disappearing into the earth. This allows the trauma to finally be over. At the end of the constellation, the client feels as if a burden has been lifted.

I accompany the process of reunifying the client with the absent soul part with the following or similar sentences:

"Welcome your soul part and allow it to sink completely into you. These are important minutes now; we have the time. Breathe in and out so that you can just about hear your breath and perceive what is happening within you. Don't judge what is happening. Give everything permission. Allow this communion, this flowing together. Your soul part knows exactly where it wants to flow. It goes to the place from which it has been missing. It has been missing in every cell of your body, in every part of your soul, in every part of your aura.

"Keep breathing so that you can just about hear your breath. Breathe in, breathe out, give permission. Breathe in, breathe out, feel.

"Allow your body to move. Follow even the smallest impulse to move. Perhaps your hands and arms want to make a certain gesture or your spine wants to straighten up, or your hips want to move. You yourself are not doing anything. Your body and your soul know how to do it. You are just there, watching it happen. It happens as if by itself.

"Perhaps you feel the soul part in a certain area of your body. Perhaps it stays there for a while, perhaps it first has to overcome a barrier, a physical hardening, and only then flows on to other areas. It also remains where it was before, so it basically spreads out.

"Breathe in, breathe out, feel, let it happen.

"Allow all the feelings that might want to come. Everything is okay here ..."

Even in the first few minutes of this ritual, something essential and astonishing happens. There is often a real liberation, a physical straightening, the development of a completely new attitude to life, never before experienced. Some clients feel as if they have been reborn.

The union with the lost soul part takes several minutes in the initial phase, but continues over many days and weeks until it finally leads to a permanent wholeness. Then, nothing is missing. The person becomes healthy.

At the end of the session, I give the client instructions on how to support this process of flowing together in a daily meditative exercise by repeating the bowl ritual and allowing it to develop further. It requires ten to twenty minutes a day. This morning ritual is important for the client to accompany and strengthen the healing process with his or her own consciousness.

With the soul part, clients often gain qualities that were previously no longer available to them. Through the integration of childlike soul parts, for example, clients often feel playful impulses in the days and weeks that follow or suddenly become adventurous and daring again.

Therapeutically guided fantasy journeys are not suitable for children, adolescents or acutely psychotic people and are contraindicated in such cases, as the risk of re-traumatisation is too great. The adult self-concept required for this is not yet developed or is weakened by the psychosis.

But with Healing Voices, a passive integration of a lost soul part is also possible in these cases.

## The support of Healing Voices

Therapeutically guided fantasy journeys are also contraindicated in cases of severe trauma or if the energy of the perpetrator is still present. In these cases, I ask the shamanic energies of Healing Voices to take healing action. As a rule, they clear the energetic field of any perpetrator energy, release the soul part from the trauma situation and guide it to the client.

The conscious integration then takes place again with the receiving ritual (bowl ritual), in which the client forms both hands into a bowl. The healer symbolically places the soul part in this bowl. Further integration then takes place in a similar way to that described above: "Welcome your soul part and allow it to sink completely into you. These are important minutes now; we have the time. Breathe in and out ..."

For children, adolescents and acutely psychotic people, Healing Voices is the method of choice for reintegrating a part of the soul that has been left behind. The receiving ritual described above is not necessary in these cases and cannot be carried out. The children are usually not present in the constellation due to their age and would also be overwhelmed by performing the ritual. Acutely psychotic patients are often in a closed psychiatric ward and are therefore not present during the constellation. Typically, the constellation for acutely psychotic patients is initiated and accompanied by their parents.

The way in which the shamanic healing powers integrate a lost soul part is impressive. In the constellation, the medium can be seen releasing the soul part from the trauma and slowly and gently guiding it towards the client. The tones and chants become higher and softer. When the soul part has reached the client, the shamanic healing powers connect the soul part energetically with the client.

159

They often make undulating or spiralling movements with their hands in the client's energy field and accompany the further merging with chants and melodies, sometimes also with primordial, empowering words.

## Case studies:

### The burden – Birth trauma
A caesarean section has to be performed because of obstructed labour. This is a trauma for the mother and the child – it was not certain whether or how the child would survive. A part of the child's soul freezes in this trauma.

In adulthood, the client feels that something is missing. She feels burdened and is therefore unable to make decisions about her professional future.

### Without a word – Separation from the mother
A baby is wiped clean, measured and weighed by the midwife shortly after birth. Meanwhile, the mother is wheeled out into the corridor to prepare the delivery room for the next birth. The separation of mother and child only lasts around seven minutes. Despite the brevity of the separation trauma, a trauma shutdown occurs in the baby. A part of the baby's soul remains trapped in the trauma.

As a result, the following symptoms appear in the first years of life: loud crying and struggling when being dropped off at nursery or in other separation situations. Speech development is significantly delayed. At the age of four, the child still does not speak.

### Migraine – Loss of the father
A father is dying. His eight-year-old daughter stands alone at his deathbed. The world closes in on her in the face of impending loss. She does not want to experience her father's death and withdraws into herself.

In adulthood, the withdrawal manifests itself in severe episodes of migraine that recur over decades and become unbearable over time.

## 2. Personal trauma in a previous life

**Therapeutic intervention:**

- Liberation from trauma freeze of the souls of the people affected at the time
- Unification of the lost soul part with the client

Every human being has many previous incarnations. If you have suffered a fatal trauma in one of these lives or have lost a loved one through a stroke of fate (trauma of loss), the unresolved feelings of this trauma can cross the energetic boundary to your current incarnation, emerge in the present emotional world and severely disrupt the course of your current life. Often a part of the soul remains in the trauma of the previous life and is missing in the present life.

In this area too, the symptom constellation is an indispensable diagnostic tool. It can be used in detective work to uncover what actually happened at the time. It also forms the framework for the shamanic healing that is always necessary at the conclusion of the constellation.

As with every symptom constellation, I start by setting up the following three positions: the client, the problem/symptom/ illness and the message it conveys. Once the information from these positions has been communicated, the next step is the four-column test.

### First positions of the incarnation constellation

If the four-column test shows that the causal energetic stress can be traced back to a trauma in a previous incarnation, the symptom constellation now becomes an incarnation constellation. I always bring the following additional positions into play:

- The person who the client was in that past life
- The trauma
- The perpetrator (this position does not exist in the case of natural disasters or illness)
- The loved one (only in cases of loss trauma, if the deadly aggression of the perpetrator or a natural disaster was directed against a loved one)
- The boundary (between the previous incarnation and the present life)
- The present life

I explain these positions to the client in detail.

### Position: The person the client was in that past life

I set up this position so that the client has a counterpart and a point of reference in the area of the past life.

I have deliberately chosen to name this position as above because there is a difference between the client in the present life and the person he or she was in the previous life. The two are not identical. That is why I insist on using this formulation throughout the constellation. This is because therapeutic work with past lives is about a clear differentiation between the present life and the past life. The exact designation of this position serves to reinforce this differentiation.

### Position: The Trauma

If the energetic cause of a problem lies in a previous incarnation, there is usually a severe trauma as the trigger. The 'Trauma' position in the constellation provides the first clues as to what sort of trauma was involved.

### Position: The Perpetrator

In the case of man-made trauma, there is always a perpetrator. This position provides information about the perpetrator. As the vast majority of perpetrators in the constellations are male, I will use the masculine form for the position of the perpetrator in the following. In practice, there are also female perpetrators. However, this occurs much less frequently in the constellations. In case of doubt, you can also find this out by placing the test positions 'Male' and 'Female' next to the 'Perpetrator' position.

If the cause of the trauma was an illness, an accident or a natural disaster, there are no perpetrators. This is also indicated by this position. The representative of the 'Perpetrator' position collapses or moves away and has the feeling of dissolving and not belonging.

### Position: The loved one

I only set up this position if the fatal trauma is not directed against the person the client used to be, but against a loved one. In such a case, however, this position is of central importance, because the original trauma is the loss of this person. The consequence is the emotional separation triggered by the early death.

The loved one often shows the typical sensations of fatal trauma: pain, suffering, agony or simply the feeling of being dead.

### Position: The Boundary

There is always an energetic boundary between the previous incarnation and the present life. However, it is often weak and cannot really fulfil the function of a boundary. Emotional energies can fluctuate freely between incarnations. The client senses something in the present but does not know where the feeling comes from. There is no obvious reason for it in the present life.

It is important to know whether the boundary is weak. Because then strengthening this boundary is part of the subsequent healing process.

### Position: The present life

The client has a present life. That's why you can also assign a position to it. I always find it interesting what the present life has to say about the current situation. At the beginning, it usually shows a defensive reaction against the influence from the previous life because it feels disturbed by it. It is also important to know how the present life is doing as the healing movement progresses. Normally, we do not stop until the representative of the 'Present life' position is feeling at ease.

After I have explained these five positions to the client, I set them up. To do this, I choose an area in the constellation room that is clearly separated from the centre where the client is standing.

The statements made by the representatives of these new positions provide clues as to what happened in the previous life. Three types of trauma are usually revealed:

1. A fatal trauma that ended the life of the person the client used to be.

2. A trauma that has ended the life of one or more loved ones. In this case, the original trauma that is causing the current symptoms is a trauma of loss suffered by the person the client used to be induced by the loss of one or more loved ones.

3. A trauma inflicted on other people by the person the client used to be. In this case, he or she is the perpetrator (most people have lived both the victim side and the perpetrator side in their previous incarnations).

The first two types of trauma can be a man-made trauma with one or more perpetrators or a trauma caused by illness, accident, a natural disaster or, in rare cases, an attack by a predatory animal. An attack by a predatory animal has very rarely occurred in the constellations I have led so far.

I therefore do not test for this possibility regularly, but only when the statements from the positions suggest this possibility. In these cases, I introduce the test position 'Attack by an animal' and proceed accordingly where the correlation is positive. Large animals such as lions, tigers, crocodiles, monitor lizards or even poisonous snakes are likely predators.

The third type of trauma, where the person who was the client at the time was the perpetrator, is by its very nature a man-made trauma.

### Procedure for man-made trauma

In man-made, fatal trauma that ended the life of the person the client used to be or the life of loved ones, the 'Perpetrator' position typically indicates a violent impact on who the client used to be or on the loved one. Typical actions include beating, strangulation, torture and so on. Or the perpetrator shows the typical movements of a paid executioner, such as pulling up a rope or striking downwards with a sword.

The more you can find out about the situation and what was happening, the better it is for the healing movement you are aiming for.

### The lone offender

The next question that arises is: Is it a single perpetrator or a system of multiple perpetrators?

To answer this question, test positions are assigned to two or three other possible perpetrators. In the case of a single perpetrator, the other perpetrators move away or collapse as an indication that they do not exist in the established system. They do not feel they belong.

In this case, we know that it was a lone perpetrator. This raises the question of the motive for the murder. The following motives mainly come into question: robbery, revenge, jealousy, greed, sexually motivated murder or madness. I set up these motives as test positions one after the other and develop the constellation depending on which motive for the murder is revealed.

In the case of robbery, sexually motivated murder or madness, there is no need to find out more. The perpetrator whose motivation was robbery or sexual gratification wants to cover up his crime by means of murder. The madman chooses his victims at random without any further background. There is nothing more to understand in these cases. Enough is known.

With revenge, jealousy and greed, there are usually other people involved. Depending on the situation, it may make sense to do further research here by getting other people to take up positions in the constellation.

## Perpetrator systems

If there were multiple perpetrators, 'Perpetrator 2' and 'Perpetrator 3' remain prominent in the field. They often indicate that they are hierarchically superior to 'Perpetrator 1', who was positioned first. In this case, they are superiors who gave orders to the perpetrators at the scene of the crime.

In such cases I try to show the chain of command up to the top of the hierarchical perpetrator system, as the aggression and negative energy in the system often emanate most strongly from the hierarchically high-ranking perpetrators, especially the commander-in-chief.

To get more information about this, I also set up a fourth, fifth and sixth perpetrator. The commander-in-chief (who can also be a woman) is usually the same as the fifth or sixth offender. He typically radiates the most aggression and negativity.

Up to this point, it is not yet known which perpetrator system is involved. In principle, all places and all times throughout human history can be considered for past lives. So, the detective work continues.

In the vast majority of cases, the person the client used to be was not the sole victim of the perpetrator system. For the subsequent healing movement, it is often important to also represent the other victims in the constellation. That is why I set up two or three other victims, representing perhaps many more, hundreds or even thousands. The other victims usually show very similar feelings to those of the client at the time.

The next question is: Was some religion the driving force behind the system of perpetrators or was it a secular system of rulers? There are many examples of both possibilities in history.

In order to answer this question, I set up the test position 'Religion'. This does not refer to a specific religion. I set this position up slightly apart from the perpetrator system. If religion plays a leading role, this is indicated by this position. Typically, it then shows an aggressive connection to the event. Or it withdraws, uninvolved.

## Religion-driven perpetrator systems

If a religion proves to be the driving force behind the perpetrator system, the next question is, which religion is involved?

To answer this question, I set up the most common religions until one particular religion shows a clear involvement. In many constellations, the Catholic Church shows up as the driving force. Therefore, I usually start with the Catholic Church as the first test position. If the Catholic Church shows no connection, I test other Christian denominations, Islam, Judaism, Hinduism and Buddhism. Most of the time you will find a match with one of these religions. If not, you have to look further and follow the clues from the constellation. I often ask the client whether a religion or a geographical area intuitively comes to mind.

Typically, the highest-ranking perpetrator (commander-in-chief) shows a close connection to the religion that has tested positive.

Religiously driven perpetrator systems torture and kill in order to maintain or increase the power and influence of a particular faith group.

## Special positions: The Goddess and the Healing Powers

If the Catholic Church or another Christian church was the driving force in the perpetrator system involved, then there is a special aspect, especially if the fate of the person the client used to be turns out to be part of the genocide of the followers of indigenous nature-based belief systems, i.e. witch hunts.

At this point, I need to expand a little. For centuries, the Catholic Church waged war against the native religions in the newly conquered territories. The old values and attitudes were demonised. People who still adhered to the old belief systems were tortured and murdered. Women and men who had ancient healing and herbal knowledge and continued to practise it were particularly at risk. They were singled out for persecution and murdered as witches or sorcerers.

Many indigenous religions were matriarchal in character and taught a completely different world view, diametrically opposed to Catholic dogma. This world view had a generally positive attitude towards life and saw human beings in deep unity with the planet, with Mother Earth. The earth was regarded as sacred. The body, as part of the earth, was also sacred. Physical love was therefore also sacred in any form (as long as it did not harm anyone). The fruits of love – the children – were the most sacred and were accorded the fullest support of the entire community.

The people who lived in the matriarchal societies with nature-based religions had the knowledge that they were always surrounded by energetic healing powers. They also knew how to honour and invite these healing forces in so that they could start healing.

Destroying the matriarchal, holistic world view and erasing it from people's consciousness was the aim of the aggressive Christian denominations, above all the Catholic Church, which castigated the body, demonised sexuality and regarded women as a fundamental evil.

The aim was therefore not only to murder these people, but also to eradicate the old healing knowledge and the world view that underpinned it.

In order to find out whether the past life trauma apparent in the present case has this background, I recommend to the client that we set up a position for the 'Healing power of the person the client used to be'. As a rule, this position indicates that this healing power exists. Often it manifests itself as bent, broken or suppressed.

Next, if the client agrees, I recommend setting up another position for their 'Personal healing power in the present life'. Most clients are very interested in this, as they often come from healing professions or have felt a more or less pronounced calling to be a healer for a long time. Sometimes they have already done further training in this direction, but feel blocked from taking the next professional steps.

The 'Healing power of the client in the present life' very often exhibits the same sensations as the 'Healing power of the person the client used to be', especially weakness and suppression. These positions show very clearly how energies and feelings from a previous incarnation can be reflected in the present life.

Many people associate the positive attitude to life of the original matriarchal religions described above with the 'Goddess' concept. In order to represent this positive life principle in the constellation and to find out whether it could play a role in the client's healing, I now recommend to the client that we also set up the Goddess as a position. If the client agrees, I place the Goddess in the area of the boundary between the incarnations. As a rule, the Goddess also shows suppression, sometimes to the point of complete extinction. The representative of the Goddess in the constellation often stands bent over or sinks to the floor.

This is an expression of the fact that, through the genocide of millions of dissenters, the Catholic Church has actually succeeded in disempowering the positive life principle of the Goddess in society, or at least in the energy field of the client. This still has an effect today. In the constellations, you can see that the aggression of the perpetrators is actually still active.

Seeing all this in its unvarnished truth has a healing power in itself. Truth heals. But the session is not yet over, the Healing Voices have not yet begun to do their work. That will come a little later.

### Secular perpetrator systems

If the position 'Religion' withdraws in the initial test as being uninvolved, you know that the perpetrator system is secular. It is thus a dictatorship, an emperor or kingdom or another ruling system, e.g. ancient Rome, ancient Egypt, the Inca Empire and so on. There are many possibilities. Here too, as in any other constellation situation, you as the constellator must not be prejudiced. You must always realise that you know nothing and allow yourself to be informed by the constellation as it progresses.

At this point, I sometimes ask the client whether any dictatorship or other ruling power or even a time or country intuitively comes to mind. If this is the case, I begin further testing with the possibility suggested by the client. Sometimes a client says "I see a dry, hot country". Of course, this can apply to many places.

On several occasions, however, this statement was a reference to ancient Egypt and a pharaoh as ruler. I take such references on board and use them as a guide for the next test position.

If there is no clue at the moment, I work my way towards the truth by setting up orientating positions, such as 'Dictatorship' (Stalin, Hitler, Franco etc.), empire, kingdom, ancient Rome, ancient Egypt. Or I set up continents and then countries to get a pertinent clue.

The constellator must (as always) be precise in defining these orientating positions. I remember a constellation of a previous incarnation in which 'Religion' did not test positive and none of the above-mentioned orientating positions registered a connection, not even 'Kingdom'. I was about to give up and said to the client that we were not getting anywhere, perhaps because this information was not necessary for healing. This had never happened to me before, but I really didn't know what to do next. Then the client said that it could also be a queen. In the end, it turned out that the most senior perpetrator was an English queen from a past century.

So even the difference between 'kingdom' and 'queendom' can prove decisive. It was indeed not a king, but a queen.

Secular perpetrator systems torture and kill in order to maintain or extend the power of the ruler or a ruling clique.

**The soul part**

If the constellation of the previous incarnation has progressed to this point (i.e. the main features of what happened are now known), I bring another, extremely important position into play. As a rule, the unresolved trauma of a previous incarnation involves a part of the client's soul that should have come over into the present life but has remained in the trauma of the previous life or is energetically frozen there.

It is important to know whether this soul part exists in the previous life. Because if it does exist, one of the tasks of further healing treatment is to find a way to bring it across the boundary into the present life so that the client can consciously integrate it.

Basically, I have never experienced that this soul part did not exist. But because you are never safe from surprises and you can never form an opinion beforehand as to how a position will turn out, I define this position as follows: 'Part of the client's soul (client's first name) that may be frozen in past life trauma'.

As a rule, this part of the soul sticks closely to the person the client used to be and has very similar feelings to them, such as deep sadness, horror, pain or the sensation of being dead.

### The effect of the detective work

Knowing the background to the trauma in a previous incarnation and being aware of the circumstances often brings about a healing movement. In order to bring this healing movement to light, I do an intermediate check at this point. In the constellation, I enquire about the state of mind of the corresponding representatives or, in individual therapy, I step into the position of the symptom, the illness or the problem, into the position of the message and, of course, into the position of the client.

Often, the symptom has already reduced its activity or ceased altogether, the illness has already retreated a few steps and the messages are satisfied with what has been set up in the previous life. The reaction of the messages is also important at this point. If something important is still missing, then the messages will show a search reaction or will see an additional person in the past life who should be considered as part of the healing but has not yet been set up.

In this case, the constellator has to make modifications. Perhaps the most important perpetrator has not yet been named and set up as the commander-in-chief, or a child is missing from the person who was the client at the time, if she was pregnant or left small children behind at the time of the trauma. These are just examples; it could be anything. The constellator should be guided by intuition and the clues from the constellation.

When the past-life-trauma is fully seen and understood, the client often shows relief and feels more positive energy.

These improvements are triggered by the fact that the client knows what happened and is aware of who was involved. The client also recognises how his or her symptom or illness is connected to this past life. Above all, however, the client sees the part of the soul that should have come over into the current life, but is still trapped in that trauma where it often still suffers excessively.

Knowing all this has a healing effect. The expansion of the client's consciousness plays an important role in the healing process. However, this is not enough to completely heal the unresolved trauma. Full liberation has not yet occurred in this phase. The problem is not yet completely solved, the way forward is not yet clear.

This has to do with the fact that the soul of the person who was the client at the time and also the soul part of the client are still frozen in the trauma. The souls of any other victims are also still suffering in the trauma freeze. In addition, the perpetrators are still energetically active.

The symptoms and problems may already show a tendency to improve at this point in the constellation, the atmosphere in the system may already feel partially cleansed, but the state of mind of the souls of those affected at that time remains unchanged. Their burdensome feelings are still in the system and prevent the full healing process.

Our human consciousness has no influence on the state of mind of those affected at that time. We as humans do not have this power. Gaining more detailed knowledge of the circumstances and background of the trauma does not enable us to liberate the souls of those who experienced the trauma personally.

In addition, the boundary between incarnations, which is actually there to protect, is still weak and permeable to the feelings of horror, grief, fear and aggression. It is as if the trauma is still happening. It is not over yet.

Now is the time for Healing Voices. Because the shamanic energies can very well initiate further healing developments.

### Healing Voices in a past life

The shamanic treatment with Healing Voices is the central healing impulse for an unresolved trauma in a past life. The client, who has so far observed the constellation from the outside, places him or herself in his/her position. In a group constellation, the representative sits down and the client takes up the position. Once there, the client must first orientate him/herself spatially so that he/she knows where the other positions are in relation to him/her. Only then does the shamanic healing begin.

In individual therapy, the client also takes his/her place in the constellation, which, like all other positions, is marked with a piece of paper on the floor. Once there, he/she orients him/herself in the geometry of the constellation. I help by briefly standing in the most important positions. Only then does the shamanic healing begin.

In the online constellation, which is common in my work, clients who are sitting in front of a computer somewhere in the world, imagine that they are standing in their place in the constellation. I help the client to do this by guiding them inwardly to this place. To do this, I ask clients to close their eyes and guide them with the following or similar words: "Imagine you are standing in a large room or a wide field, your symptom has already retreated a little and is about two metres to your right. A few metres behind you is the boundary to your previous life. Behind it is the person you were back then, still suffering from the trauma. Your soul part, which should actually have come over into this life, is also still over there and is suffering, the perpetrators are further back..."

Shamanic healing only begins once the client has orientated themselves spatially.

At this point the client is already informed about Healing Voices, has received all the necessary information from me and has expressly agreed to the shamanic treatment.

Nevertheless, I find it important that the client receives a short briefing now that he or she is standing in the constellation and waiting for Healing Voices to begin. The following formulation has proved successful:

"You can close your eyes if you wish and just listen and focus on what is going on inside. But you can equally open your eyes now or later and see what is happening in the room during the shamanic healing, or switch between the two modes, depending on what is more comfortable for you at the time.

"If the healing voices become loud and aggressive, don't be afraid. You are on the safe side. You have my assurance in this regard. Even though I will be working as a medium for the next few minutes, I am not in a trance but am very much present and aware of everything that is going on. So you are not alone in this experience.

"After working with the perpetrators, the Healing Voices often work with the victims. In this case, you may hear plaintive or mournful tones. After this, the voices become softer and often more melodic. In this phase, the Healers can also come to your domain to provide you with energetic support, perhaps to help you let go of a residual burden. Is that okay for you?"

If the client agrees to this as well, the shamanic healing begins. As described in detail above, Healing Voices first work with the perpetrators, disempower them and destroy them energetically. They then typically release the soul of the person who was the client at the time and the souls of all other victims from the trauma freeze.

As a special feature of working with past lives, Healing Voices strengthen the boundary between incarnations. The precise way in which this happens varies greatly and depends on the individual case. Sometimes it happens covertly and I, as a medium, don't notice it at all. At other times, the shamanic healing powers work intensively for several minutes on strengthening and sealing, sometimes even embellishing this boundary.

At an unspecified point in time, the Healers carefully and gently bring the part of the client's soul that was frozen in the trauma across the boundary to the client and connect the two energetically.

However, this step must also be carried out in the client's consciousness. It is not enough for Healing Voices to prepare the way for union in the client's unconscious. The client must take this step consciously. This is achieved with the bowl ritual, which significantly supports the union with the lost soul part. This ritual is basically the same as described in the chapter on personal trauma in the present life on page 156. The intensity of the 'healing explosion' that occurs is also quite comparable. The union with the lost part of the soul, the becoming whole, takes several minutes in the initial phase, but continues over many days and weeks until it finally leads to a lasting wholeness.

The point at which I introduce the bowl ritual depends on the constellation setting. If the client is present and physically in place in the constellation during the shamanic healing, I will conduct the bowl ritual at the point at which Healing Voices bring the soul part into the immediate vicinity of the client. To do this, I step out of the Healers' position, pause the shamanic healing and conduct the bowl ritual. When the ritual is underway, the client consciously welcomes the soul part and the energetic confluence has already begun, I continue to work as a medium. The shamanic healing continues. Furthermore, Healing Voices support the confluence of the soul energies, perhaps cleanse the client's energy field, harmonise the entire field of the system and so on.

In online constellations, where the client is sitting somewhere in the world in front of a laptop, I will only conduct the bowl ritual after the Healing Voices have done their work. This is more appropriate for this setting and has the same liberating effect.

Shamanic healing takes about ten to twenty minutes, rarely longer than half an hour. But at some point, the work of Healing Voices is done.

I then step out of the Healers' position and sit down for a minute or two, during which the energy of what has happened resonates. I then ask the representatives in the various system positions to report how they are feeling after the healing. This information is important for clients, expands their awareness and informs them about the current (healed) situation:

The boundary is strong and no longer allows any disruptive energies to pass through. The perpetrators are disempowered and have disappeared. The person the client used to be is released from the trauma. Their soul can go its own way or reconnect with other people from whom it was separated by the trauma. The lost part of the soul has crossed the boundary and is in the process of integrating itself into the client's personality. The client is already feeling the effects. Something fundamental has changed. The symptom, illness or problem has lost energy or has already completely dissipated energetically.

The healing movement has begun internally, but will continue to develop over the coming weeks and months. On a physical level, the body cells need a certain amount of time to adjust to the new energetic situation. The improvement in symptoms may start soon, perhaps even be noticeable at the moment, but it often takes days and weeks for the full healing effect to develop.

So that the client can support the healing movement that has now begun consciously, I recommend that he/she does a morning exercise for three to four weeks in which he/she remembers the healed situation in the constellation and repeats the bowl ritual in order to continue experiencing and supporting the confluence with the soul part.

**Case studies:**

### Rage against men – The slave hunters

In a previous life, a woman loses her husband, children and other relatives to slave hunters. The slaves are beaten. Many are killed. The woman is filled with vengeful aggression against the perpetrators. But the perpetrators are long gone.

Revenge aggression overcomes the energetic boundary to the present life.

In the present life, the woman is overcome by uncontrolled aggression against men, especially against men with whom she enters into a relationship. All relationships break down.

### Autoaggressive disease – The execution

In ancient Rome, a woman is captured by the Roman emperor's henchmen and executed by sword. The aggression of revenge against the emperor and the other perpetrators transcends the boundaries of present-day life.

In the present life, this unconscious aggression triggers an auto-aggressive disease of the thyroid gland and also uncontrollable outbursts of anger which the client cannot control and of which she does not know the origin.

### The emotional wall – Murder in Spain

A Frenchman leaves his wife and children to fight with the International Brigades against the Franco regime in the Spanish Civil War. He is captured, tortured and murdered. He preferred to fight for his political convictions in a war waged in a foreign state. The abandonment of his family weighs on his soul as guilt which, together with the horror and suffering of torture and murder, is imprinted on his energy field. These emotional energies cross the boundary into his next incarnation.

In his current life, the client suffers from an insurmountable detachment towards his children.

## Procedure in the case of fateful trauma

If the 'Perpetrator' position indicates that there is no perpetrator, then it is a non-man-made trauma, in other words a purely fateful event in which no human being had a hand. There are many possibilities: an illness, an accident, a natural disaster such as storm, flood, earthquake, avalanche, volcanic eruption, fire, lightning strike and so on, also (but rarely) an attack by an animal.

The procedure in the constellation is also aimed at finding out as much as possible about what happened. Even if there are no perpetrators here, there is still detective work to be done.

Again, the trauma was fatal, either for the person the client used to be or for one or more loved ones. First, I test the major categories and start with the most common. I start with the test position 'Illness'. If this item is clearly linked to the trauma, you know that an illness was the cause of death.

I then test whether it was an epidemic, because in this case there are also other victims that should be added to complete the picture. In the case of epidemics, I go on to test which epidemics they were – plague, cholera, typhoid, Spanish flu and so on.

If the 'Epidemic' position tests negative, I know that it was a disease that only affected one person. I do not carry out any further tests in this case because the specific disease involved is not important for healing.

If 'Illness' tests negative, I proceed to the 'Accident' position and, if necessary, continue with the natural disasters until the nature of the trauma has been established. Sometimes there are clues from the positions or the client has inner images of the catastrophe in his/her mind's eye, e.g. water or fire. Sometimes, as the constellation facilitator, I see a scene that tells me which catastrophe I should test for next.

The further procedure is basically the same as for the man-made trauma described above, with the exception that there are no perpetrators.

When everything important has been set up in the constellation, the feeling can occasionally arise that something is still missing. It is often the position which I call 'Message of the symptom or illness' that provides this information. In these cases, it is important to remember that the system may still be looking for a perpetrator, even though there is none.

This may have something to do with the fact that people also seek an explanation for a fateful event, a causal connection. But fateful events such as an earthquake or a volcanic eruption are not the fault of any human agent. Fate is stronger than mankind.

We find it difficult to deal with senseless fate. That's why we often look for someone to blame. Perhaps we have done something wrong ourselves or someone else has angered the gods with their behaviour or even God himself is to blame because he did not prevent the earthquake or the flood. However, the search for a perpetrator that does not exist is a disruptive factor in the system.

So if, in the case of a non-man-made trauma in a previous incarnation, the impression arises in this phase of the constellation that the picture is not yet complete, I set up the test position 'Fate'. If this position shows a clear connection to the event, the energy in the system changes. Because now the client and everyone else involved realises that no one is to blame. Fate is stronger than we humans. The search for a perpetrator can now also be abandoned in the unconscious. Now everyone, including the client, is exonerated. This has a calming effect on the entire system.

The shamanic healing forces that I invite in the final phase of the constellation do not need to concern themselves with the energy of the perpetrator, as it does not exist. Otherwise, the process of shamanic healing is very similar to that described above for unresolved man-made trauma, including the bowl ritual for the conscious integration of the soul part left behind.

## Case studies:

### Exhaustion – The plague
In the Middle Ages, a woman dies of plague along with thousands of others in her town. In the most intense suffering of the dying process, her soul becomes locked in the trauma freeze. The deep exhaustion overcomes the boundary to the present incarnation. In the present life, she feels a deep fatigue that makes it impossible for her to lead a full private life in addition to her job.

### Depression – The volcanic eruption
In a previous incarnation, a man loses his beloved wife in a volcanic eruption. He cannot get over this loss and remains buried in grief for the rest of his life.
The grief is so strong that it succeeds in overcoming the energetic boundary to the present life. In the present life, the client feels depressed and isolated even as a young man and considers suicide.

### Ataxia – The earthquake
A woman loses her beloved husband in an earthquake. There are many other victims. She is unable to move on from the grief arising from the trauma of loss, is lost for words and becomes rigidified. She can never break free from this emotional numbness.
The grief, the numbness and the silencing are so strong that they overcome the boundary to the current incarnation. In her current life, the client suffers from a severe neurological disorder that renders her unable to move around without a walking aid. Recently, she has also developed a worsening speech disorder. She can hardly get a word out.

### Procedure if the client was a perpetrator

Many people have had incarnations on both sides of the victim/perpetrator divide.

If the person who the client was at the time was a perpetrator, the perpetrator energy is already clearly evident in the position of the person who the client used to be at the time.

In these cases, it is not a question of guilt that still needs to be borne or atoned for in the present life. Rather, the aggression and arrogance of the person who the client was back then, as well as the grief and pain of the victims, can cross the boundary into the present life, become perceptible in the present and can be the cause of symptoms, illnesses and problems. However, this has nothing to do with relevant guilt or punishment in the present life, but is a well-known, energetic occurrence as a result of an unresolved trauma in a previous life.

In these cases, I go on to set up the victims in the constellation. I usually take three victim positions as being representative for possibly many more, sometimes hundreds or even thousands. The victims usually show the typical feelings of victims who are locked in the trauma freeze. Depending on the individual case, co-perpetrators can also be set up.

Next, I establish a part of the client's soul that is frozen in the trauma. This part of the soul also exists in these cases. It often shows the emotions of suffering, pain and oppression. There is an inner moral authority in perpetrators, a part of the soul that suffers from the fact that this person has become a perpetrator. The perpetrator has to defy this inner authority, suppress this part of his soul, in order to become so hard and heartless that he can murder other people.

If this inner authority is a part of the soul that should have come over into the present life but is frozen in the trauma, then the client will be missing it in this life.

The further procedure is very similar to that of man-made trauma, in which other people were the perpetrators.

Healing Voices deal with the perpetrator energy of the person who the client was at the time in the same way as with the perpetrator energy of other perpetrators. It is destroyed, the perpetrator is disempowered.

It is an unusual situation for the client to realise that he/she had become a perpetrator in a previous life, that the person he/she was then is being disempowered and energetically destroyed by shamanic healing forces and that now a dubious soul part is also coming across the boundary with the aim of becoming reintegrated. But ultimately the integration of the soul part works here just as it does in other situations. If the client knows that this soul part belongs to him/her and is nothing strange or dangerous, he/she can usually consciously invite and welcome it in the bowl ritual

**Case studies:**

### Lust for power – The (female) pharaoh

I remember one case in which the client complained about not being able to form lasting relationships and often reacting aggressively to her partners and fellow human beings in a completely unjustified way. She couldn't do anything about it.

It turned out that in a previous life she was a domineering pharaoh who had thousands of people murdered.

The desire to dominate and the claim to be untouchable had already manifested itself in her childhood and had become a problem in her relationships with her parents, siblings and teachers. Later, all her important relationships were ruined as a result.

### Sexual blockage – The nun

In the Middle Ages, a nun is member of a Catholic system of perpetrators that tortures, rapes and murders many women. She turns the women over to the Inquisition. The suffering of the victims overcomes the energetic boundary between incarnations.

In the present life, the guilt and fear of being hurt expresses itself as a sexual blockage. In intimate situations, the client feels nothing.

### Disorder – The mass murder in India

In the 19th century, during Queen Victoria's reign in India, an Englishman becomes a perpetrator by participating in mass murders as a high-ranking army officer. As a result, something is fundamentally disordered in his soul.

In his current life, the client finds it difficult to keep his home tidy. His flat is becoming increasingly cluttered. He feels powerless to do anything about it. His last girlfriend left him because of this. He cannot bring himself to receive guests any more.

## Procedure for previous lives without trauma

A symptom can also have its energetic cause in a previous in-carnation in which no trauma occurred; on the contrary, a special happiness and deep fulfilment may have prevailed. I call this the 'Golden Age syndrome'. The reason why a soul part that should have come over into the current life stays behind in such a happy incarnation is not because it is frozen in an unresolved trauma, but because of the attraction exerted by a wonderfully contented exist-ence in happiness and fulfilment. The soul part simply does not want to go into a later, burdened epoch in which the marvellous inner talents are blocked and in which the client knows nothing of the happiness and wisdom that he or she already achieved back then.

Nevertheless, this part of the soul is missing in the present life. As is so often the case, symptoms, illnesses or emerging problems indicate that something is wrong, that something is missing. In this case, it is the indication that the client should connect with the level of existence already reached. To do this, however, the client would first have to know about it.

This connection can be uncovered in a symptom constellation.

Specifically, the four-column test shows that the symptom pre-sented has to do with a previous life. However, the position 'The person the client used to be' feels itself to be in a wonderful energy, perhaps standing with arms wide open, connected to the commu-nity and the whole universe. This is a state that the healer tries to achieve in other cases in which an unresolved trauma plays a role. But here this paradisiacal state has already been reached. There is nothing to heal at this point. There is no trauma. This is indicated by the 'Trauma' position collapsing or moving away. In most cases, many other people are positively connected to the person the client was at that time in the sense of a community. These people also usually feel wonderful and have a beautiful, revitalising contact with each other.

When I saw this for the first time in a constellation, I was amazed. How could a previous incarnation lived out in this golden, paradisiacal state lead to problems and symptoms in the current incarnation? It didn't make sense at first.

But after a few minutes of letting the situation sink in, I had an idea. Perhaps there is also a part of the soul that was left behind in a previous life for whatever reason.

I set up a new position, which I called 'Soul part of the client (first name), which may have been left behind in the previous life'. This soul part did indeed exist. However, in contrast to the cases I had known until then, it was doing wonderfully well. It stood upright in joy next to the person who was the client on that occasion and felt freely connected on all sides. It did not want to go into another life in which it was suppressed or disregarded.

But it was defined as a 'Soul part of the client in the present life'. So it belonged in the current life. Its absence triggered the current symptoms.

So, a healing movement was needed to heal the symptoms. As with all other incarnation constellations, I left it to the shamanic healing powers of Healing Voices to find a way to energetically guide this part of the soul towards the client so that she could consciously integrate it. In this way the client regained access to the positive energy of the previous incarnation. The impetus that this development triggered in the client's current life was clearly felt in the weeks that followed. Her life began to realign itself in a direction that she would never have dreamed of before.

Even if such cases have been relatively rare up to now, you as the facilitator should be aware of this possibility so that you can also be helpful for such clients.

**Case study:**

### Intestinal paralysis – The Golden Age

A woman experienced a 'Golden Age' in a previous life. She was a great healer, lived with many other people in a large community, felt happy and blissfully connected to the world and the universe.

In her current life she has no connection to her healing qualities and knows nothing of the happy, fulfilled existence in her previous life. She lives an entirely normal life, has an entirely normal job, has entirely normal problems. But one day she falls ill with a mysterious illness. She repeatedly suffers intestinal blockages, some of which are life-threatening. The doctors cannot find a physical cause. It is as if her life as a whole is coming to a standstill. She is missing the part of her soul that should have come over to the present life, but, under the given circumstances, apparently prefers to stay in the previous life. However, she absolutely needs it for the next phase of her life.

### 3. Trauma in the present family

The present family is the family that you have founded in the course of your life, although this definition is broad. Your own present family includes all important past and present romantic partners, whether you married them or not, whether they are living or deceased. Which romantic partners belong in the systemic sense depends on the depth of love and connection that exists in the conscious or unconscious. No human being can decide this with a pure act of will. Belonging is indicated by the fact that the loss of a partner through separation or death triggers such a strong trauma of loss that it can still have a disruptive effect on your own energy field years and decades later and cause symptoms, illnesses and problems.

Experience shows that partners to whom you were or are married or partners with whom you have or had a child are definitely included. But the circle of partners who belong to the present family is often much larger. Sometimes future romantic partners also come into the equation.

All of your own children are also part of the present family, whether living or deceased, including those who were miscarried or aborted. An unresolved trauma experienced by one's own child is always an energetic burden for the parents and can trigger symptoms of various kinds, even after a long time. This also applies to traumas experienced by children in adulthood.

If the four-column test in the symptom constellation indicates that there is a causal connection between the symptom, illness or problem and the present family, I interview the client at this point to find out who belongs to this group of people in the individual case and what traumas have occurred. I ask the client:

Are you married, in a relationship or single? Have you ever been married, engaged or had a significant romantic relationship?

Have you lost someone from this group of people through separation or death? Or has a romantic relationship been thwarted by outside influence, e.g. a parental prohibition?

How many children do you have? How many miscarriages? Have you had any abortions?

Did you lose children early? What traumas happened to your children? And so on.

Once the people who belong to the present family have been named and the traumas in this domain that the client remembers have been communicated, I next set up the 'Original trauma' position. This is defined as the trauma that energetically caused the problem, symptom or illness that the client has presented with. It must be in the domain of the present family, as this is the area which the four-column test has addressed.

The next step is to find out who exactly was involved in the original trauma. I base this on what the client tells me, ask more detailed questions if necessary and, as a test, put forward the partner or child who is most likely to be involved.

Sometimes you can guess right from the start what the trauma is and who was involved. I remember a client whose young wife had been killed in a car accident. I set up positions representing the wife and the car accident. The car accident immediately connected with the original trauma that had already been set up. This made the original trauma clear. It was the loss trauma of the client who had been widowed.

In other cases, the original trauma is not so clear. Perhaps the person involved has not yet been named as belonging because the client assumed that he or she was not important enough. Or the client has forgotten the trauma because it was too painful, or she did not consider it relevant, e.g. an early miscarriage. In these cases the facilitator has to investigate further. The original trauma must be somewhere in the present system. The four-column test has indicated this.

I remember a man who came to me because he was unlucky in love. None of the partners initially mentioned by the client showed any connection to the original trauma. He didn't have any children. But the trauma had to be somewhere.

I asked him about a childhood sweetheart. He told me that he would have liked to have got engaged at the age of 18, but that his parents had forbidden the relationship because they had not considered his girlfriend to be appropriate. The client had complied with his parents' wishes at the time. The relationship, which had barely begun, was broken off. After that, he largely forgot the story. When we set up a position for this girlfriend, she immediately showed a clear connection to the original trauma, which now turned out to be a loss trauma for both the client and the ex-girlfriend. When I set up the 'Love' position, it turned out that both are still connected in the unconscious by a great love.

Once the nature of the original trauma and the people involved have been identified and positioned, the aim is to initiate a healing process. In the case of loss traumas, where there has been an emotional separation between the client and the loved one, healing occurs through the reconnection of the two souls. This is sometimes achieved on a conscious level through Healing Sentences that are said to the other person in order to respectfully re-establish the connection. Healing Sentences are part of classical family constellations as taught by Bert Hellinger. A typical Healing Sentence spoken to a partner who died young might be: "Dear wife(husband), your death was terrible for me. I couldn't get over it for such a long time. Now I am looking at you again. The love between us remains."

Sometimes it works, the feelings flow, something is released inside. However, this requires that the other person, the soul of the prematurely deceased partner, is willing and able to engage in emotional dialogue. In the case of violent forms of death such as a car accident, however, it is possible that the soul is still locked in the trauma freeze of the accident, feels as if it is lying dead on the road and cannot hear or feel anything else.

In these cases, the Healing Sentences are not sufficient for healing to take place, even if they are meant quite sincerely. The emotional separation is still present and the trauma therefore remains unresolved.

Only shamanic healing can help here. In the case of the man described above, who lost his beloved wife in a car accident, this was precisely the case. The woman was locked in the trauma freeze. I asked Healing Voices to work beneficially in the man's system. The shamanic healing powers were able to release the woman's soul from the trauma freeze. In the end, the two of them stood closely entwined and were connected with great love and joy. The emotional separation caused by death had been nullified. It was a love that lasted beyond death.

In the second case described above of the man who was not allowed to marry his girlfriend by his parents, Healing Sentences did not bring any emotional reaction from the client either. He faced his girlfriend from back then. Love stood strongly between them and wanted to unite them both. The girlfriend reached out her hand, ready to approach and reconnect. But the man was defensive, emotionally uninvolved and couldn't understand on an intellectual level why this girlfriend should still be so important to him after thirty years.

At this point I had the idea that, as is often seen with other loss traumas, a part of the man's soul could still be frozen in the loss trauma. I set up this part of the soul as a position. It stood next to the loss trauma in deep sadness. The unification with this soul part succeeded here by means of Healing Voices. It could now also be consciously accomplished by the client in the bowl ritual. This opened his heart, which he had closed at the behest of his parents.

At last he could feel the grief he had suppressed for so many years. It was now able to flow away. Now he could look his girlfriend in the eye. In the end, these two were also closely connected with love and joy.

The background and the events of an unresolved trauma in the present family can take different and diverse forms. The procedures applied in the healing process are guided by this. Healing Voices has also made a whole new level of healing possible here and is now also an integral part of therapy in this area.

**Case studies:**

### Marital problems – The abortion
A married woman aborts a child because the doctor advises it, as the pregnancy occurred despite the IUD. The couple do not grieve for the child.
As a result, the relationship with her husband is disturbed. The intimacy is lost. Years later, the couple are on the verge of divorce.

### Unfulfilled desire for a partner – Sudden death
A woman loses her beloved husband to a heart attack at work. She is unable to say goodbye to him.
Many years later, she desperately wants a new relationship. But as soon as a new man tries to enter her life, she shies away. The now repressed pain of losing her first husband is still too great. Unconsciously, she is afraid of experiencing something similar with a new partner.

### Tinnitus – Separation from a loved one
Six months before a planned marriage, the woman falls in love with another man. She is completely fulfilled when she is with

him. Nevertheless, she marries the fiancé for practical reasons. This ends her relationship with her lover.

Twenty-five years later, she develops persistent tinnitus. No therapy helps. The tinnitus is there to remind the client of the romantic relationship between her and the lover. She can no longer ignore it.

## 4. Trauma in previous generations of the family

### General information

Bert Hellinger performed a great service to humanity in uncovering the enormous importance of unresolved traumas in earlier generations of the family of origin as the cause of many physical and mental symptoms and illnesses, as well as many relationship problems, and also in developing a method with which many family burdens can be resolved – the systemic family constellation.

I honour Bert Hellinger as one of my greatest teachers. Without him, I would never have been able to do the work I do today. Family constellations were my starting point thirty years ago. Even today, far more than half of my symptom constellations result in a family constellation.

In 1993, Gunthard Weber published the first book on Bert Hellinger's family constellations, *Love's Hidden Symmetry* (German title: *Zweierlei Glück*). After that, Bert Hellinger himself and many other authors wrote dozens of books about it. They have been translated into many languages. My own book *Weiterbildung in Systemaufstellungen*, in which I summarise the most important principles of constellation work, was published in German in 2003.

Decades have passed since then. A lot has changed. We have all learnt more in the meantime. Hellinger himself has developed other types of constellations over the years. Practitioners around the world have changed and developed family constellations based on their experiences and different backgrounds. Inspired by my experience, my knowledge as a doctor and as a philosophical thinker, I too have added some new elements to the classic family constellation and developed the Symptom Constellation that I now offer to people from all over the world. The most important new element is the connection with Healing Voices and the extended healing possibilities that arise from this.

Fixed components of the classical family constellation such as Healing Sentences, on the other hand, have become less important in the Symptom Constellation. Sometimes, they are still indispensable today. Mostly, however, they play a subordinate role. In classical family constellations, Healing Sentences were used in a respectful ritual in an attempt to return the family burden to the parent or grandparent concerned. According to the systemic orders of the family formulated by Hellinger, the ancestors had to deal with this themselves. This is basically still the case today. The orders of love still apply.

Through the shamanic healing energies of Healing Voices, however, it is now also possible to free the souls of those people who actually experienced the trauma at the time from the stressful, energetic consequences. This dissolves the energetic burden in the entire system. The parents and grandparents still have to find their own way of dealing with the newly resolved situation. The child and grandchild have nothing to do with this. But if the original trauma has also been resolved in the souls of those affected at the time, it simply no longer makes sense to carry a burden through the generations. It falls away by itself or can finally be actively let go. The result is a relief in the entire system that can be felt on several generational levels.

A conscious handing back by means of Healing Sentences is often no longer necessary for healing in the case of energetic burdens that are dissolved by themselves, but is sometimes helpful as a supplement.

However, I would like to emphasise at this point that even today you should not attempt to do a constellation to heal your own parents or grandparents. That would be presumptuous and would never lead to the desired outcome. But in the case of a constellation for one's own personal problem or a problem of one's own children, in the course of a Healing Voices treatment, which is carried out as part of a symptom constellation, there is regularly also an energetic relief at the level of the parents, grandparents and more distant ancestors, which they themselves have to deal with. As a descendant, you have no influence on this. Nevertheless, I like the idea that, as a symptom carrier, your own healing also has a healing effect on many other family members. You are not alone with the symptom and you are not alone with the healing.

The second major innovation that I have introduced into family constellations is a clearly structured approach that considerably eases the detective work tracking down the original trauma behind the problem the client is presenting with. The realisation that this original trauma in the family system always exists when it is indicated in the four-column test has inspired me to always set up the still unknown original trauma as a position and thus have a reference point to find out to which generation and to which family member it belongs. With this reference point, the original trauma can usually be identified, even if it has never been discussed in the family.

In the past, the idea was that you could end the constellation when you had prepared the next step for the client. Today I get to the bottom of the matter and usually do not stop until I have identified the original trauma where the energetic burden began. I also set up positions for the affected people who were involved with the trauma at the time, paving the way for Healing Voices to free them from the trauma. The affected people, deceased or living, must be positioned in the constellation so that the shamanic healing powers can release them from the trauma. This allows the client to consciously experience the healing and see what happens to the previously affected person in the course of the healing. The expansion of the client's consciousness plays an important role at this point.

A third, very important area has undergone a transformation in the last twenty years. This is the way in which we deal with the perpetrators and the victims. In the early days of constellation work, nobody had begun to consciously integrate shamanic healing powers into family constellations. They may have been present and effective to a certain degree. Everyone who has experienced many constellations is familiar with the phenomenon that something happens in the constellation as if by itself in the direction of healing. But at that time, all you could do with stubborn perpetrators who held on to the negative energy and murderous aggression was to show them the door and make it clear that they had forfeited their right to remain in the family system. I remember that this intervention was often the only way to bring peace into the system.

Some perpetrators felt remorse even without the intervention of the facilitator, sank to their knees in front of the victims and wept bitterly over their actions. Some of these perpetrators then lay down quietly next to the victims, if the victims allowed this. In some constellations conducted by Bert Hellinger himself, the perpetrators and victims lay on the floor and moved closer to each other in a spirit of peace. I also experienced this later in my constellations. Many people subsequently concluded from this that, as a constellation facilitator, you should try to keep the perpetrators in the system and work towards integrating them, because otherwise there can be no good solution. Sometimes I still hear this opinion from constellation facilitators today. In my experience, however, it is fundamentally wrong. No facilitator should make it their job to keep a perpetrator in the system.

The reason why I am now so sure of this is because I have worked with Healing Voices for decades. They always have an effect on the perpetrators if the latter have been assigned a position. I have seen only two reactions in terms of healing: on the one hand, the destruction and disempowerment of those perpetrators who cannot be separated from the negative, murderous energy; on the other hand, the deep remorse of the perpetrators who can be separated from the negative energy by Healing Voices, very similar to what sometimes happens spontaneously in classical family constellations without a conscious invitation from shamanic forces.

However, what is necessary for healing at the level of the perpetrator is not decided by the constellation facilitator, but happens without his/her intention and without his/her intervention. The facilitator is neither a prosecutor nor a judge. After all, it is precisely this impartiality that enables the facilitator to successfully lead a constellation or to be a medium for Healing Voices.

Once the negative, murderous energy has been destroyed, Healing Voices can free the victims from the trauma freeze. The direct energetic work with the victims is also another difference to the classic family constellation. Back then, the facilitator was content when the victims lay calmly and peacefully on the floor. This gave the whole system a peaceful feeling. It was not thought that the souls of the victims could be energetically freed from the violent trauma so that they could go the way they were supposed to after death, free from trauma feelings. But this is exactly what happens when Healing Voices work in perpetrator-victim fields. The souls of the victims are released from the agony of death, become emotionally alive, feel a great liberation and open up to the path that lies ahead of them.

The trauma is now history and finally consigned to the past. It leaves the client's energy field. The path to healing is open.

## Detailed procedure for a family constellation as part of a Symptom Constellation

If the four-column test indicates that the family of origin is causally related to the problem the client has presented with, the symptom constellation becomes a family constellation at this point.

One of the most important tasks of family constellations is to find the original trauma in the family system and thus create the conditions and framework for the healing movements described above through Healing Voices. The following procedure has proved successful:

### The interview

I do not conduct the interview about the family of origin until after the four-column test and not at the beginning of the session, because only now is it clear that the energetic cause lies in the family of origin.

Firstly, I ask some basic questions about the family, such as:

"How many brothers and sisters do you have? Are there any siblings who died early, were miscarried or aborted, as far as you know? Are your parents still alive? Are they together or separated?"

Next, I ask more in detail about the side that the four-column test has indicated, either the maternal side (left arm) or the paternal side (right arm). If the response is from the maternal line, there is no need to ask for more background about the father and his ancestors. This is a relief. It saves time and effort, because it is unnecessary to memorise the paternal family tree plus traumas if it is not about that side of the family tree. In this case, you concentrate on the mother:

"How many siblings does your mum have? Are there any siblings of the mother who died early, were miscarried or aborted? Are there one or more traumas in your mother's family? For example, was the grandfather or someone else in the war?" And so on.

Sometimes the four-column test indicates that both lines are involved in the energetic background of the problem. This means that there are two original traumas, one on the maternal side and one on the paternal side. In this case you have a lot of work ahead of you, because you now have the task of working with both sides and doing two constellations in one session in order to solve the problem, the symptom or the illness. Of course, you can also do this in two separate sessions. But why wait if the client's receptive state allows you to deal with both in one session.

### The first positions

Once the information has been gathered as far as possible and the client has told you everything important, it is necessary to find the original trauma and the generational level at which it happened. To do this, I set up the 'Original trauma' position, usually a little away from the centre. The 'Original trauma' position is defined as the trauma that is the cause of the current problem, symptom or illness.

Next, in this case, I assign a position to the client's mother (we'll stay on the mother's side for the sake of simplicity).

The mother is usually also affected by the original trauma or directly involved if the trauma happened to her. More often, however, the trauma belongs to an even earlier generation.

To find this out, I assign positions to the mother's parents, the grandfather and the grandmother. Depending on the information from these positions, there are clues as to which of these two lines the burden stems from. You may have to go back several generations and assign positions to the great-grandparents or great-great-grandparents until you find a generation that no longer shows any relationship to the original trauma.

Most of the time, you find the trauma already on the level of the parents, grandparents or great-grandparents. At this point, there is usually already a suspicion or a clear indication of which family member or members were involved in the trauma.

If, during the interview, the client has reported a trauma in the maternal line that you already suspect is the original trauma, you can set up this trauma as a test early on to see whether it actually has a connection to the original trauma or not. If this connection does not emerge, you continue to work with the unknown.

In principle, it can be any type of trauma. There are thousands of examples. One could fill entire books with them, which has indeed already been done.

The further procedure is individual and depends on the situation and the information coming out of the constellation. This opens up a wide field in which you as the constellation facilitator let yourself be guided by your intuition and trust in your perceptive faculties.

Nevertheless, I would like to describe some typical situations in which a structured approach has proven its worth. These are by no means instructions for action, but purely examples of how this can be done.

### War traumas

In the case of war trauma, for example, a certain approach has proved successful. A common case is the involvement of a grandfather in a war trauma. It can also be the father, the great-grandfather or another family member. For the sake of simplicity, I will choose the grandfather as the family member involved.

War traumas were often concealed. Sometimes a client doesn't even know whether the grandfather was in the war or not. In this case, we work with the unknown.

At a certain point in the constellation, all we know is that the grandfather has something to do with the still hidden original trauma. We do not yet know which trauma it is and in what way the grandfather was involved.

If the client tells me that grandfather was a soldier in the Second World War, I set up 'Second World War' as a test position at this point to ascertain whether the original trauma occurred during the Second World War. If the information from the position confirms this to be the case, the detective journey can continue. The most common war traumas that appear in constellations are war crimes, defined as the murder of unarmed prisoners or civilians.

To test whether it is actually a war crime, the next thing I do is set up victims, usually three victim positions representing often many more. The constellation tells you whether these victims exist in the system or not. The positions clearly indicate this. If the victims feel that they belong (i.e. they do not move away, but remain in place and show their suffering), then you know that it was a war crime because, by definition, the victims in the constellation are murdered people, in contrast to those who died on the battlefield. Death on the battlefield does not constitute murder and is therefore not considered a war crime.

At this point, it is often not yet clear what role the grandfather played in the war crime in question. He could be a perpetrator or a victim or a contemporary witness, which can be a trauma in itself. The grandfather's reaction to the victims provides the first clues:

If the grandfather shows clear aggression towards the victims, he was obviously among the perpetrators. If he shows compassion and sadness towards the victims, he was usually not with the perpetrators.

However, the reactions of the grandparent can vary greatly in this situation. Often there is a feeling of not being involved or an inner aggression and anger that has no direction. In these cases, the grandfather's role in the war crime is still uncertain; he may still be a perpetrator or just a witness.

To find that out, the next step is to position the perpetrators, the murderers. Someone has committed the crime. Here, too, I start with three perpetrator positions and then expand to five or six, until the highest-ranking perpetrator (i.e. the one who usually displays the most aggression and the most negativity) is part of the constellation, for example, Hitler for Nazi crimes, Franco for war crimes committed by the Spanish dictatorship.

If the relevant perpetrators are positioned in the perpetrator system, the grandfather's reaction is interesting. If he shows a friendly affinity with the perpetrators or, for example, gives Hitler the one-arm salute, then we know that the grandfather at least sympathised with the perpetrator system and supported it. Direct participation in the crime cannot be deduced from this.

If the grandfather vehemently rejects any involvement, so vehemently that one may conclude from this that he was involved in a secret way, I set up the 'Guilt' position as a further aid in the detective work. If 'Guilt' indicates a connection to the grandfather, in whole or in part, we know that he was involved as a perpetrator in some way, even if he shows no clear aggression towards the victims. He may have denounced people to the Nazis, knowing full well what would happen to them.

This can be checked in the constellation by setting up the test position 'Betrayal'. If it shows a connection to the grandfather, you know that he was a traitor and thus became a perpetrator.

The situation is quite different if the grandfather exhibits aggression and anger towards the perpetrators at the moment they are set up. Then he usually harbours revenge aggression against the perpetrators. This is a clear sign that he was not a perpetrator, but was one of the compassionate people who were on the side of the victims. He may have witnessed innocent, defenceless people being attacked or murdered, but had no way of protecting or avenging the victims. Perhaps the grandfather had the urge to help the victims and take action against the perpetrators, but suppressed this urge because he himself was trapped and helpless (e.g. Holocaust survivors) or out of fear of being shot himself (e.g. soldiers who witnessed war crimes).

It is also often the case that the grandfather came on the scene too late because the murders had already taken place, but he saw the bodies and could do nothing about it.

Many of our ancestors experienced such situations in the First and Second World Wars. Those who survived the war or the Holocaust internalised the revenge aggression and took it home with them. Even if they wanted to forget what had happened so that they could somehow continue to live 'normally', the energy of revenge remained there and circulated within them. In this way, it found its way into the family energy field of those affected and was passed on to descendants over several generations via epigenetic processes. The result is autoaggressive and autoimmune diseases in the descendants.

This is why revenge aggression is a major issue in family constellations. Every family constellation facilitator should have detailed knowledge of revenge aggression mechanisms, because they have a major impact on families over generations.

There are basically two types of aggression. The first type is the aggression of a perpetrator. It is directed at other people who have done nothing to provoke the assailant's aggression. The second type is defensive aggression. It can later become revenge aggression.

Defensive aggression is a healthy reaction to an attack. Everyone defends themselves when someone attacks them. We protect life and limb – our own and that of the people we love. We mobilise all our strength to defend lives.

Defence aggression is directed at the aggressor, the perpetrator. If you cannot show defensive aggression because you are too weak, are somehow trapped, are afraid for your own life or arrive too late, then you have a problem. The perpetrators have disappeared and can no longer be found. In this case, defence aggression becomes revenge aggression.

You want to take revenge, to bring your aggression to bear on the target, to take revenge on the perpetrators. This is a primordial process. If you are unable to catch up with the perpetrators, the energy of revenge cannot take effect. It remains stuck in your own energy field and in your own body as a destructive force. It goes round and round within you, lacking a target.

Revenge energy follows the law of conservation of energy, which states that energy cannot dissipate into nothing, but can only transform itself by releasing energy, i.e. by doing what comes naturally. Revenge aggression must therefore do something. That is in its nature.

If it gets trapped inside an individual because the perpetrators it wants to pounce on are unavailable, it begins to turn against that individual's body and soul over time. The consequences are auto-aggressive diseases, e.g. cancer, rheumatism, polyarthritis, multiple sclerosis, polymyalgia, skin rashes, allergies, depression with suicidal tendencies and much more besides.

Revenge aggression can already develop when we witness other, innocent people being murdered, even if we have no personal relationship with the victims. However, the fact that it has an effect over several generations may indicate that the grandfather (to stay with our present example) had a closer relationship with at least one victim, e.g. a relationship of love. During the Second World War, it was very common for German soldiers to have love affairs with women from an occupied country. If, for example, the woman was murdered in a mass execution as part of a punitive action following a partisan attack, revenge aggression arose among these soldiers. It was directed against the German perpetrators, i.e. against their own people, but often could not be acted out. These men brought their revenge aggression home with them after the war.

In order to find out in a constellation whether the grandfather had such a personal relationship with one of the victims in the given case, I set up the test position 'Victim who had a personal relationship with the grandfather'. If this position actually exists, it has a major impact. It is often a loving relationship with a woman. In this case, you can often see the grandfather's grief rising up behind the revenge aggression. This reveals the deeper connections.

As soon as it becomes clear in the constellation that the grandfather is filled with revenge aggression and that the perpetrators are the target of the revenge aggression, he already feels relieved: "At last someone understands what happened to me".

At the same time, a weakening of the autoaggressive illness or suicidal threat can often be seen in the constellation. Simply by knowing the connections, by knowing what has happened, a healing process is already initiated.

Once the original trauma has been identified and it is clear which family member was involved and in what way, and all other related positions have been set up, we investigate the effects of these connections on the client and on the symptom. The message of the symptom is also consulted in order to be sure that nothing has been overlooked. Because if something or someone is still missing, this will be indicated by the 'Message of the symptom' position.

The next step is shamanic work with Healing Voices, as described in detail above.

**Case studies:**

**Fear – The war crime**
An Englishman serves as a soldier in the British army during the Boer War and becomes a perpetrator by participating in the killing of civilians, women and children. He unconsciously takes the fear experienced by the victims back to England in his energy field. He later marries and emigrates to a distant country. His great-grandson takes up a profession as an assistant in a psychiatric clinic. Whenever he treats clients suffering from the

consequences of a violent crime, he is overcome by an inexplicable fear that weighs heavily on him. He is on the verge of burnout.

## Allergic asthma – The gas attack

The lover of an Austrian soldier dies during a gas attack in the First World War. The soldier is filled with vengeful aggression against the perpetrators. But the perpetrators are the leaders of his own nation. They cannot be brought to justice. The revenge aggression is unconsciously passed down through the generations in the energy field of the family.

The great-granddaughter develops allergic asthma (auto-aggressive disease) as a child, which leads to emphysema with shortness of breath in middle age. She can only manage everyday life with a constant supply of oxygen. (Shortness of breath is the leading symptom of gas attacks)

## Compulsive washing – Betrayal to the Nazis

A man denounces people to the Gestapo, knowing full well as a convinced Nazi that they will be murdered as a result. After the war, he manages to cover up his treachery. But in his family's energy field, the guilt and stigma are unconsciously passed on to the next generation. As an adult woman, his granddaughter develops a compulsion to wash that lasts for decades.

## Anorexia nervosa – The mass shooting

A man actively participates in mass shootings under the Greek military dictatorship. When the dictatorship falls, he flees to South Africa, where his uncle lives. The man lives a completely normal life there, never returns to Greece and is never prosecuted.

But the revenge aggression of the victims is in his energy field and is passed on energetically in his family. A granddaughter develops a life-threatening anorexia.

**Early loss**

Many original traumas concern the early loss of family members who were often not adequately mourned. In order not to be reminded of the deep pain, their surviving relatives marginalised and forgot them. There is a strong taboo in the families affected against talking about the trauma. But the grief is buried deep in the unconscious, even if in later generations no one knows what actually happened.

The trauma of loss may have been triggered by an early death through illness or accident, by suicide or also by the murder of a family member, e.g. in the Holocaust, or by other acts of violence.

Revenge aggression plays a major role in violent deaths. In 'victim families', it is often hidden behind grief, lethargy and depression. But it is hidden somewhere and can also lead to auto-aggressive diseases and even suicide over multiple generations.

If the loss trauma has been kept secret in the depths of the family and the client knows nothing about it as a result, a structured, detective-like approach is helpful in the constellation.

The fact that a loss trauma is involved often becomes apparent early on in the constellation when great grief becomes apparent or someone is 'searching for the dead'. Typical signs of this are when the representative of the client or the symptom kneels on the floor and searches with their hand on the floor for something or someone or makes a digging motion or when a position looks upwards as if into the sky and searches with their eyes for someone up there. However, the clues can take many forms.

Here, too, a position is assigned to the original trauma. Through setting up the generations step by step, you try to find the affected generational level and the family members who died or were murdered at an early age.

Sometimes you have to go back to the great-grandparents or even further. I can remember constellations for indigenous clients in North America in which we had to assign positions to the ancestors who were murdered in a mid-19th-century genocide in order to find a solution. Here, too, it was significant that we had a reference point in the constellation with the 'Original trauma' position.

But it is not always a matter of murder, war crimes and genocides. The early loss of family members through natural causes of death such as illness, sudden infant death syndrome or accidents can also cause severe traumas of loss that can burden multiple generations. Of course, you try to find out by asking specific questions whether such traumas are known. But here too, much is repressed and forgotten. Nevertheless, the original trauma must be found so that the marginalised family member can be brought back into the consciousness of the client and the family, as well as ensuring that targeted healing through Healing Voices is possible later on.

The death of a former spouse in the parents', grandparents' or great-grandparents' generation is often due to illness or childbirth. In the latter case, the wife (as well as the child, if it also died at birth) is often stuck in the trauma freeze, while the bereaved husband (father, grandfather, great-grandfather) is frozen in the trauma of loss. His heart is shut down by the pain. In such cases, the blockage at heart level can be passed down through generations to the client, making a fulfilling loving relationship impossible.

In such cases, there is no need to assign positions to perpetrators because there are none. Healing Voices can therefore work directly with the souls of people who have died prematurely, free them from the trauma freeze of early death and release their loved ones from the trauma of loss. As a result, the loved ones become aware of each other again and come together in love and joy. The child is also freed from the isolation of the trauma and typically now lies peacefully and calmly in the mother's arms.

This image of family members connected in love (e.g. the nuclear family with great-grandparents and child) is deeply healing for the client. Grief can be allowed to flow. The heart can open across the generations. Joy and loving closeness are now possible.

Another common example is the death of multiple children in infancy or early childhood. A hundred years ago, this was still a common occurrence in Central Europe. Ten or fifteen children per family were not uncommon. Medical help was poor to non-existent. In some constellations, for example, the great-grandmother and great-grandfather are full of grief in the trauma of loss, while four or five deceased children lie isolated and suffering on the floor in front of them. Here too, Healing Voices is often the only way to achieve a truly profound and sustainable energetic healing in the system.

**Case studies:**

### Cardiac arrhythmia – Death of a loved one

A man fights as an American soldier in Asia during the Second World War. His unit liberates an island from Japanese occupation. On the island, he falls in love with a local woman and enters into a relationship with her. Weeks later, she is killed in a Japanese bombing raid. He buries the pain of losing his lover deep inside. After the war, he tries to forget it all, marries and has children.

But the heartache remains in his energy field and is unconsciously passed on in the family.

The man's granddaughter develops cardiac arrhythmia and an inexplicable, excessive sadness at the very moment she falls in love.

### Heartache – The broken engagement

At the age of 20, a young woman gets engaged to her boyfriend, with whom she is deeply in love. The young woman's parents do not think the relationship is appropriate and exert pressure on their daughter to the point where she gives in and breaks off the engagement. From then onwards, she closes her heart to love and life in general. She no longer sees any great meaning in life, but marries another man years later.

The 'closed heart' and the feeling that life is pointless and no longer has any meaning persists in the energy field over the generations and resurfaces in the granddaughter. She has recurring heartaches and feels fundamentally depressed and uninvolved in life.

**At risk of suicide – Death in childbirth**

At the end of the nineteenth century in Italy, a young woman dies giving birth to her child. The child also dies. The woman's husband is unable to cope. The grief is too strong. He just wants to get away, start again, leave everything behind. He emigrates to the USA. Beforehand, however, his family arranges a new engagement. After a few months, the seventeen-year-old bride travels to the USA to join her husband. However, the grief has travelled across the Atlantic and carries over in the family's energy field to the man's granddaughter. After a separation, she falls seriously ill with depression and wants to take her own life.

## Outlook

Once the original trauma has been resolved, the connecting and sustaining energies become active and take over. They create a connection to the healthy source of life from which the body cells are sustained. Now that the blockages have been removed, the sustaining energies can realign and renew themselves. Healing also takes place on an emotional level. In the constellation, people who belong together are connected, approach each other, embrace each other and radiate peace and deep joy.

The life energy is liberated and shows strong, positive effects. The client's energy field is harmonised. The healthy connections with the energy fields of other people, of nature and of the greater whole are revitalised. Health and a sprightly, joyful attitude to life are restored.

The healing effect of symptom constellations in combination with Healing Voices is powerful and far-reaching. These two energy medicine methods will revolutionise medicine in the coming decades. To achieve this, however, it is necessary that many people, doctors, therapists, alternative practitioners, system constellators and other qualified people are trained in the shamanic healing method known as Healing Voices.

I present the concept for this training programme below.

### Training in Healing Voices Rainbow®

In order to protect the training for Healing Voices healers and to ensure that this method is only carried out by competent, qualified therapists, I have registered 'Healing Voices Rainbow®' as a trade mark. The term 'Healing Voices' cannot be protected because it is too general and many therapists around the world already offer healing work with other methods under this label. So I looked for an extension of the term. I decided on 'Rainbow' a few years ago when I stepped out of the house after an online workshop for Healing Voices and beheld an unimaginably large, crystal-clear, double rainbow that spanned the whole horizon. The special feature of this rainbow, apart from its size and clarity, was the fact that it retained the same intensity for an hour. The people in our village still remember that day well. They sat outside their houses and marvelled.

At this moment, I realised that Rainbow was the right extension. The training is therefore called Training in Healing Voices Rainbow®. When you read this name on a practice sign, you can be sure that you are putting yourself in skilled hands.

The training programme lasts several years and is divided into four consecutive training units, each of which takes graduates to the next level of competence.

## Contents of the training

The focus of the training is on preparing students for the task of working as a medium for Healing Voices. This primarily means working on one's shadow side, the proactive detection of disruptive energies in the student's energy field, for example fearful or aggressive energies or generally blocking energies. (see chapter The Medium starting on page 121)

The training also centres on freeing students from disruptive influences of the ego such as arrogance or false modesty.

The shadow work and the liberation from ego influences take place during the training period in numerous symptom constellations in combination with Healing Voices. From the very beginning, the students experience many case studies in which they repeatedly explore the method to be learnt in 'live' application with themselves and other participants.

The principles and procedures of shamanic work are taught in detail as early as the basic training programme.

The principles and strategies of symptom constellations are also an essential part of the advanced Master's programme. At the highest level, the Trainer module, the principles of training and supervision are added to the mix.

## Structure of the training

- **Healing Voices Rainbow® Practitioner**
  Basic level
  Expertise: Healing Voices in individual therapy (without symptom constellation)
  Duration: 2 years, 4 x 3 days per year, total duration 24 days

- **Healing Voices Rainbow® Healer**
  Expertise: Healing Voices in individual and group therapy (without symptom constellation)
  Duration: 2 years, 4 x 3 days per year, total duration 24 days

- **Healing Voices Rainbow® Master**
  Expertise: Healing Voices in symptom constellations, collective healing, individual and group therapy
  Duration: 2 years (1st year 6 x 3 days – 2nd year 5 x 3 days + 5 days workshop to conclude the Master class), total duration 38 days

- **Healing Voices Rainbow® Trainer**
  Expertise: Trainer in Healing Voices in all modalities, Healing Voices in symptom constellations, collective healing, individual and group therapy, supervision
  Duration: 2 years (1st year 6 x 3 days – 2nd year 5 x 3 days + 5 days workshop as trainer conclusion), total duration 38 days

The training in Healing Voices Rainbow® therefore takes several years, depending on which qualification you are aiming for. The training is an intensive time for all students, during which they experience accelerated personal development. This is both an opportunity and a challenge. It takes courage and a declared willingness to recognise and heal the shadow areas in one's own unconscious and the inhibiting influences of the ego. This involves working on yourself. In the course of time, you get to know all the connections you have as a human being. In the process, new ground is broken again and again. It is an adventurous journey towards finding yourself.

The effort and commitment are worth it, because during the training, students gain deep insights into the human condition in all its primal reasons and possibilities. They develop the ability to act as a medium for the powerful shamanic healing powers of Healing Voices. At the same time, they become part of a growing global community of people who are acquiring and applying extraordinary healing skills.

Every qualified Healing Voices Rainbow® healer will be able to make a powerful contribution to the healing of many people. Satisfaction, joy and success are the inevitable outcome of this contribution.

It is a wonderful feeling to live and work in the certainty that, with Healing Voices, we are always surrounded by powerful healing forces, wherever we are and in whatever life situation we find ourselves. Healing Voices are always with us and are also willing to help and heal us, if only we have the knowledge how to invite them in mindfully and without making any demand on them.

The future is healing! It begins in this very moment.

## Appendix

### Further case studies

The case studies in this book illustrate how symptoms, illnesses and problems can develop as a result of burdensome trauma energies in a person's energy field. Knowing these mechanisms is the prerequisite for being able to heal with energy medicine.

The case studies do not describe the healing process after a symptom constellation or shamanic healing. Of course, as a doctor, systemic constellator and shamanic healer, I know from experience that the vast majority of clients benefit significantly from my work and many even experience complete healing.

But a statistical survey in the form of a study conducted professionally over months and years has not yet been carried out in the field of Symptom Constellations combined with Healing Voices. I therefore see no point in publishing 'success stories', of which I am obviously aware, but which do not really allow the reader to get a clear picture of the enormous healing power of this work. For that, you would also need to know how often it hasn't helped.

This book can contribute to future scientific studies that measure the enormous success of the combination of Symptom Constellations and Healing Voices in verifiable statistics.

Nevertheless, the case studies in this book are of great value in their abundance because they open our eyes to the major role that the human energy field plays in the development of illnesses, symptoms and general life problems.

The key points of the case studies have been modified in such a way that they cannot be assigned to a specific case. Most of the examples have several or even many individual cases in the background and thus represent an essence from a pool of experience. Nevertheless, they describe typical cases as they occur every day in my practice or in my online therapies with clients from all over the world. They are therefore quite normal, everyday cases.

## Case studies – Family of origin

### Suicidal behaviour – Rape of the great-great-grandmother
Towards the end of the 19th century, a woman is raped by several men on a ship on the Baltic Sea and dies two days later as a result.

Her husband only finds out later what has happened. He is filled with revenge aggression. But the perpetrators are not caught. The revenge aggression is passed down the generations to the great-great-granddaughter, who falls ill with depression at the age of 15 and tries to take her own life.

### Outbursts of anger – A Nazi grandfather
A German man works in a weapons factory during the Nazi era. In order to become a foreman, he joins the NSDAP. He mistreats forced labourers from Poland and the Czech Republic. Many of them die of malnutrition or direct murder in the camps where they are held or in the factory. The revenge aggression of the victims continues in the family system of this perpetrator right down to his granddaughter. She suffers from an underlying anger that repeatedly erupts and makes her life difficult.

### Failed marriage – Rape of the grandmother
A woman is raped. She doesn't talk about it. The anger and revenge aggression towards the perpetrator turn into aggression and rejection of everything male, which is felt above all by the man who later becomes her husband. This woman's daughter is also raped by a stranger at a young age. She can only talk about it on her deathbed. She too represses the revenge aggression against the perpetrator into the unconscious, where it is likewise transformed into a rejection of everything male, which in this case is also felt above all by the husband. The rejection of masculinity and the feeling of having to protect oneself from men is passed down through the generations.

219

The granddaughter still harbours this energy, which makes a fulfilling relationship impossible. She cannot experience intimacy and deep emotional connection. Her marriage is at risk of breaking down.

**Psychosis with risk of suicide – The Irish Potato Famine**
A young woman emigrates from Ireland to the USA in the 19th century. The reason is the famine in Ireland, in which several family members have died. She harbours revenge aggression against the English, who she believes deliberately exacerbated the consequences of the famine in order to decimate the Irish population. The revenge aggression is passed down through the generations and leads to a psychosis in the great-great-grandson with the risk of suicide. In his psychosis, he is searching for perpetrators whom he must destroy in order to save innocent people.

**Uncontrolled outbursts of rage – Murder of children**
A man murders indigenous children in 19th-century America, an act carried out together with other perpetrators. This happens within a framework approved and desired by the highest political level in the USA.
The revenge aggression of the indigenous relatives of the victims continues in this man's family for generations. This man's great-great-grandson still unconsciously harbours this aggression. It repeatedly erupts in fits of rage that cannot be controlled.

**Rage against men – Undiscovered murder**
A man is murdered, and his killer escapes undetected. The victim's wife is filled with revenge aggression, but doesn't know what to do with it. Revenge aggression is passed down through generations in the female line and is directed against everything male, especially husbands.

The granddaughter of the murdered man's wife becomes aggressive towards her husband for no reason. He has no idea what he has done to deserve his wife's accusations and anger. He turns away from her in disillusionment.

## Outbursts of rage – A spy in the ranks
A man serves in the American army during the Second World War. He has access to secret information about potential bombing targets in Britain, which he reveals to the Germans for money and out of sympathy for Nazi ideology. His spying activities are never discovered.

But the revenge aggression of the British bombing victims reaches his personal energy field, from which the aggressive energy is passed down through generations in the family system. His grandson develops inexplicable fits of rage. The people around him are afraid of him. He doesn't understand this, because he actually sees himself as a peaceful person who strives for balance. But the outbursts of rage become more frequent.

## Nightmares – Murder of the great-aunt
A young woman is raped and murdered on her way home. The murderer is never identified. After some time, the woman's family stops talking about her and her fate to prevent the pain from coming up again and again. Her sister also buries the pain somewhere inside. She later marries and has children. Her children learn nothing about the murder. But the victim's fear and the perpetrator's aggression are still in the family's energy field. A granddaughter of the murdered woman's sister develops nightmares as a child, from which she wakes up screaming. The nightmares get worse in her youth. She dreams of someone who wants to murder her. Frightened, she hardly dares to go back to sleep.

### Fear – Murder of the great-great-grandfather

A man doesn't come home from work. He has fallen victim to a violent crime. His body is never found. The family remains in the dark. The man remains missing.

The fear of the perpetrator's aggression is passed down through the generations. A great-great-grandson of the man develops an anxiety disorder in his early youth. He is constantly afraid that something terrible will happen. If someone opens a door unexpectedly, he flinches. He absents himself from school.

### Fear of loss – Grandmother dies in childbirth

A woman dies giving birth to a child. The child also dies. The husband tries to suppress the pain. Later, he will never discuss this event again. The second wife knows about it, but the family do not talk about it. The husband's grief and fear enter the family's energy field and are passed on to later generations.

A granddaughter develops inexplicable fears of loss as soon as she enters into a relationship with a man. At the same time, she is afraid of intimacy. The tension between these two fears makes a fulfilling, lasting relationship impossible.

### Unfulfilled desire for a partner – Rape

A woman is raped by Russian soldiers in the final days of the Second World War. During this period, she witnesses many other women in her neighbourhood being murdered.

The fear and revenge aggression towards the perpetrators haunt her throughout her life. These feelings are passed on in the family's energy field.

Her great-granddaughter has an inexplicable fear of men. At the same time, she feels anger welling up inside her in intimate situations. She wants a life partner, but this wish goes unfulfilled. She has the feeling that she is hardly noticed by men.

## Depression – Enslavement of ancestors

In the 19th century, slave hunters invade an African village and enslave many people, driving them in chains to the coast and shipping them off to America.

The suffering and grief continue in the family systems of the victims. Over 100 years later, a descendant of one of the victims is carrying the energetic burdens in her energy field. She falls ill with depression, can no longer cope with life and develops suicidal thoughts.

## The separation – Massacre in Africa

An Englishman joins the British army in the 19th century and is posted to an African colony. There he takes an active part in a massacre of the local population. He never talks about it at home. He and his comrades are even celebrated as heroes for the successes of his regiment.

The massacre permanently separates the victims from their loved ones. The energy of separation continues in this man's energy field for generations. His seven great-grandsons and great-granddaughters have had no contact for years. They no longer talk to each other and blame each other for this. They live in isolation, scattered around the world.

## Blockage of a fulfilled life – Betrayal to the Nazis

A man denounces fellow citizens to the Nazis during the Second World War. They are murdered. The traitor manages to keep his treachery a secret even after the war. But the suffering of the victims is in his energy field and is passed on energetically through the generations. His great-grandson carries a blockage that prevents him from living a fulfilled life. He repeatedly experiences separation and loss.

## Abdominal pain – Rape of a great-aunt

A three-year-old girl is raped by a landowner. She dies as a result. The child's parents cover up for the landowner because they are financially dependent on him. The girl's sister is traumatised by the incident.

The sister's granddaughter develops abdominal cramps during puberty, which recur for decades. Recently the pain has become unbearable.

## Case studies – The present family

### The dilemma – Abortion
A woman aborts a child at a young age. She doesn't tell the child's father because she has just separated from him.

Decades later, when she is happily married to another man, her husband decides to move abroad for a while. He wants his wife to come with him. But she can't make up her mind. She feels as if she would have to leave an important person back home. Even though she doesn't know who that might be, she is stuck in this dilemma.

### Breaking off a relationship with her son – Separation from a first boyfriend
A young woman ends a relationship with her first boyfriend with whom she had been together for four years. She lost one of his children at an early stage of pregnancy.

Decades later, having just gone through a divorce, her adult son breaks off his relationship with her. She can no longer get in touch with him. He is entangled with the miscarried child from the previous relationship.

### Relationship disorder with daughter – A plane crash
A married man loses his life in a plane crash. He is only forty years old. The family's grief for him is unredeemed. The wife finds no emotional connection to her husband, as his soul is frozen in the sudden, violent trauma. The unresolved trauma also threatens to damage relationships between the other family members.

Ten years later, the widow's relationship with their daughter, now grown up, deteriorates. She denies her mother any contact with the grandchildren.

### Unruly children – Sudden death of a mother from an abdominal aneurysm

A young, married woman with two school-age children dies suddenly and unexpectedly from an abdominal aneurysm. Her soul freezes in this sudden death situation. The grieving family cannot find an emotional connection with her. The grief and pain remain unrelieved.

During puberty, both children become difficult to control and mentally unstable. Their school performance deteriorates. The father no longer knows what to do with them.

### Diverticulitis – Feelings of guilt due to accidental death of fiancé

A man dies in a car accident.

Although it is clear that another motorist was to blame for the accident, the man's fiancée blames herself because she had a premonition before the journey and believes that she did not do enough to dissuade her fiancé from driving.

The trauma of loss and the conflict of guilt lead to the development of recurrent diverticulitis many years later. The internal wound of loss has not yet healed and continues to fester.

### The brake on life – Death of a first beloved

A six-year-old girl is close friends with the neighbour's boy, who dies at the age of five after a long illness.

Decades later, the client (the girl now grown-up) realises that she is not making progress in several areas of her life. She feels fundamentally impeded. A part of her soul had been left behind in the trauma of losing her first love as a child.

### Polyarthritis – Abortion at the age of 18

A young woman aborts a child at the age of 18. Subsequently, she rarely thinks about it.

Five years later, she develops polyarthritis, which lasts for decades. In her mid-forties, she is in a wheelchair and continues to have joint pain. The illness is there to remind the client of her child so that she can reconnect with her child internally.

**Uncertainty – Separation from the first great love**
A young man finds the love of his life at an early age. Under pressure from his parents, he breaks off the relationship. He is twenty years old at the time.

Decades later, he is haunted by a personal insecurity that makes it impossible for him to assert himself and his rights in his personal and professional life. He did not stand up for his great love, and now he lacks the courage to stand up for himself. He is missing a part of his soul that is held back by the trauma of his youthful separation.

**Anger at the husband – Miscarriage**
A married woman suffers a miscarriage in the third month of pregnancy. She develops feelings of anger towards her husband, who did not want the child and whom she therefore blames for the miscarriage. The woman's overwhelming anger prevents her from mourning her child. Soon after, the couple divorce.

But ten years later, the woman is still sitting on her anger, which is still directed at her ex-husband and now also at their grown-up son. The relationship with the son deteriorates. He no longer wants to know anything about his mother and no longer visits her. The client suffers as a result.

Case studies – Personal trauma

## Problems with boundaries – Near-death experience of the mother

Complications occur during the birth of a child. The midwife underestimates the danger. An emergency caesarean section is performed. The woman giving birth is close to death. She has a near-death experience, has already left her body and is looking down on herself from above. The danger passes. She and the child survive.

The woman already has a seven-year-old daughter who is at school at the time of her sibling's birth and knows nothing of the events in the hospital. But her soul senses that her mother is close to death. A part of the daughter's soul freezes in this near-loss and assumes that the mother has actually died.

In adult life, the daughter has problems maintaining her boundaries with other people. There are repeated violations of boundaries to which she cannot react adequately because she is afraid of losing the relationship. The grief of the soul part locked away in the near-loss trauma plays a decisive role in the unconscious energy field. The problem with boundaries causes relationships with partners and friends to repeatedly break down.

## Fear of intimacy – Sexual abuse in a convent school

A seven-year-old girl is sexually abused by several people of both sexes in a convent school.

As a teenager and as an adult woman, the client is afraid of intimate situations and therefore prefers to be on her own. She can't stand being close to friends either. She is lonely.

## Recurrent infections over years – Dental surgery

A four-year-old boy undergoes dental surgery under general anaesthetic due to extensive tooth decay. The parents have to wait in the anteroom. The doctors refuse to allow them to stay with the child during the operation.

From school age to adulthood, the client is susceptible to a wide range of infectious diseases. He has trouble fending off germs. He is often absent from school. As a teenager, his recurrent illnesses prevent him from fulfilling his great potential as a football player.

## Repeated injuries – Circumcision

A boy is circumcised as a baby.

As a teenager (17), he repeatedly injures himself in sport. These are unusual injuries for his age group. The original trauma is repeated above all in the area of the muscles and joints. The tension in the tissue is deep-seated.

## Depression and anxiety – Violence by the father

A girl is repeatedly beaten by her father. She receives no protection from her mother. In the violent traumas, a part of her soul freezes in the torpidity of the trauma and 'stores' the fear and terror in the unconscious energy field.

As early as puberty, she feels depressed and anxious. Years later, when she is already over forty, the depression intensifies and the anxiety escalates into panic attacks.

## Blocked love – Death of two triplet brothers in the womb

A girl loses her two triplet brothers as a result of miscarriage.

During puberty and later as an adult, she feels something freeze inside her as soon as a man touches her intimately. As a result, all her couple relationships break down. Intimate touching unconsciously reminds her of the close physical togetherness with her triplet brothers and, at the same time, of the pain of separation.

### Low-energy syndrome – Lumbar puncture

At the age of seven, a girl undergoes a lumbar puncture, which she fiercely resists. She passes out for several minutes during the procedure. The memory of this defenceless exposure is stored in her energy field.

In adulthood, the client suffers sudden physical weaknesses (low-energy syndrome) that last for days and have become more frequent in recent months.

### Spinal complaints – The mother's suicide threat

As a child, a boy is exposed to his mother's suicide threats over many years. This burden weighs heavily on him.

As an adult, he develops chronic spinal pain. The painkillers barely help. The energetic burden from the childhood trauma is also too much for his spine.

### Worry about the son – Car accident during pregnancy

A woman has a car accident when she is five months pregnant. She suffers minor injuries but, for the next few days, is terrified of losing her baby. The child is born healthy at the normal due date.

The trauma of the car accident leads to the woman still being afraid years later that something bad could happen to the child. She becomes an 'overprotective mother', which severely inhibits the child's development.

### Disorder of sexual experience – Kidnapping with rape

An adult woman is kidnapped by a man and raped several times. Only after some days is she able to escape at the risk of losing her life. The perpetrator is caught and convicted.

After this trauma, the client's ability to experience sexual relations is severely impaired. Even fifteen years later, nothing has changed.

## Case studies – Past incarnation

### Anxiety – Murder in ancient Egypt
A woman is hanged by the Pharaoh's executioners in ancient Egypt, along with many others. The fear, the panic and the feeling of not being able to breathe crosses the boundary into the current incarnation.

In her present life, the woman has recurring anxiety episodes, which have escalated into panic attacks over the past couple of months. She has been admitted to the Accident and Emergency department three times during the last week.

### Pustules – Plague in the Middle Ages
In the Middle Ages, a man loses his beloved wife in an outbreak of the plague. The trauma of loss causes him to fall into a depressive agony that lasts the rest of his life.

In his current life, he develops pustules in his youth, which break out again and again over decades. They appear in the places on the body that are typical of plague.

### Unlucky in love – The witch hunt
In the Middle Ages, a woman with healing powers is hanged along with many others by the henchmen of the Catholic Church. The feeling of being a victim crosses the boundary to the present incarnation.

In the present life, the client always feels victimised in her relationships with men. She repeatedly experiences painful separations. She is unable to achieve her goal of a fulfilling, happy relationship.

### Rheumatoid arthritis – The murder of the healers
In the Middle Ages, a woman with healing powers is tortured, raped and murdered along with many other victims by the Catholic inquisition. The revenge aggression against the perpetrators crosses the boundary into the current incarnation.

In her present-day life, it manifests itself in rheumatoid arthritis (autoaggressive disease), which has persisted for many years and is difficult to treat, even with cortisone, making the client wheel-chair-bound.

### Multiple sclerosis – Execution of a non-convert
In a previous incarnation, a woman is hanged by a Muslim perpetrator system because she does not want to accept the new faith (Islam). The revenge aggression overcomes the boundary to the current incarnation, gains access to the client's energy field and manifests as multiple sclerosis (autoaggressive disease), which takes away all her strength. She can only walk a few metres.

### Fear of human closeness – The early loss of a loved one through illness
In a past life, a woman loses her beloved husband at a young age due to illness. In this trauma of loss, she freezes in grief and profound disillusionment. She can no longer enter into new relationships. She turns away from life.
This defensiveness against an intimate relationship overcomes the boundary to the current incarnation and intensifies to become a fear of any human proximity. The client lives in isolation. Her desire for social closeness to friends or even to a possible life partner is not fulfilled.

### Breast cancer with bone metastases – Murdered by the Inquisition
In the Middle Ages, a woman is tortured and murdered by the executioners of the Catholic Church. The suffering crosses the energetic boundary to the current incarnation.
In her present life, the client is diagnosed with breast cancer complicated by multiple bone metastases.

### Parkinson's disease – Murdered by the Inquisition
In the Middle Ages, a woman is tortured and murdered by the executioners of the Catholic Church. The suffering and the

revenge aggression towards the perpetrators energetically transcends the boundary to the current incarnation.

In her present life, the client falls ill with Parkinson's disease (autoaggressive disease). She becomes weaker and weaker over time.

## Separation anxiety – Murder of the mother in the Second World War

In a previous life, a Polish boy witnesses the mass shooting of civilians by German perpetrators during the Second World War. His mother is among the victims. This trauma haunts him throughout his short life.

In his present life, the child client, now four years old, lives in great fear of being separated from his current mother, who is participating in the constellation on his behalf. In separation situations, he cries until he is back in his mother's arms. Daycare and kindergarten are therefore not options.

## Panic attacks – Loss of husband and child in an epidemic

In a past life, a woman loses her beloved husband and daughter in an epidemic. She sinks into deep grief from which she cannot find her way out for the rest of her life. She withdraws from all social contact and lives as if incarcerated in an internal prison.

In her current life, the client developed panic attacks and a social phobia in early adolescence, which keeps her away from all social contacts outside her immediate family. She can no longer go to work.

## Acknowledgements:

First and foremost, I would like to thank Dr Bruno Weidlich, Chief Physician at Memmingen City Hospital, and Dr Eberhard Kalhammer, Chief Physician at Memmingen District Hospital, for providing me with such a free and collegial environment for my specialist training in internal medicine over a ten-year period. Above all, I would like to thank Dr Christian Borck, Senior Consultant of the Internal Medicine Department at Memmingen City Hospital at the time, who introduced me to psychosomatic medicine and supported me in all matters.

Special thanks are due to Dr Konrad Stauss, head physician at the Psychosomatic Clinic I, Bad Grönenbach, who introduced me to the importance of the spiritual dimension of healing. I would also like to thank Dr Jürgen Klingelhöfer, Head Physician at the Psychosomatic Clinic II, Bad Grönenbach, under whose guidance I received in-depth training in psychotherapeutic group therapy and other humanistic forms of psychotherapy.

My greatest thanks go to Bert Hellinger, who taught me family constellations and expanded my understanding of illness and healing to include the dimension of the transgenerational energy field.

I would also like to thank Dr Gunthard Weber and Prof Dr Matthias Varga von Kibéd for broadening my horizons to include further possibilities of systemic constellations.

I would especially like to thank Tacansina, the shaman who gave me my first personal healing experiences with shamanic energies. He also introduced me to the ritual of an Indigenous North American sweat lodge, where I later received Healing Voices for the first time.

Then I would like to thank fate, which took me to twenty clinics throughout Germany between the ages of 50 and 60 as part of my honorary work as a physician. This has given me a deep insight into the current situation of modern hospitals run by conventional medicine, especially at their focal points. The experience has made me realise the special value of energy medicine in the patient care of the future.

I would especially like to thank my American colleague Dr Anngwyn St. Just, who has enabled me to present Symptom Constellations in combination with Healing Voices in fourteen countries on three continents. The workshops Anngwyn and I have facilitated together in different cultures are unforgettable. Anngwyn has greatly enriched my understanding of trauma.

I would like to thank my son Ryan, who did a wonderful job editing this book. I would like to thank my daughter Melanie for the portrait photo. I would also like to thank my wife Irmgard Rosa Maria from the bottom of my heart for her support and encouragement in all areas. Irmgard has accompanied me from my first beginnings in conventional medicine through all the sometimes-turbulent phases of my professional career.

I would also like to thank Andrew Swift for translation into English and Margaret Swift for proofreading.

I would also like to thank my clients who have placed their trust in me. This book has only been possible because of the experience I have gained from working with them.

**Contact to author:**

E-Mail: karl-heinz@dr-rauscher.de

Website: https://www.dr-rauscher.de/en

Facebook: https://www.facebook.com/karlheinz.rauscher/

Youtube: https://www.youtube.com/@Dr.Rauscher

Instagram: https://www.instagram.com/karlheinzrauscher/

LinkedIn: https://www.linkedin.com/in/karl-heinz-rauscher-14999218/